KV-051-793

THE
TOPIC
OF
CANCER

WHEN THE KILLING HAS TO STOP

THE
TOPIC
OF
CANCER

WHEN THE KILLING HAS TO STOP

By

DICK RICHARDS

Kent Private Clinic, Sandwich, Kent, England

PERGAMON PRESS

OXFORD · NEW YORK · TORONTO · SYDNEY · PARIS · FRANKFURT

U.K.	Pergamon Press Ltd., Headington Hill Hall, Oxford OX3 0BW, England
U.S.A.	Pergamon Press Inc., Maxwell House, Fairview Park, Elmsford, New York 10523, U.S.A.
CANADA	Pergamon Press Canada Ltd., Suite 104, 150 Consumers Road, Willowdale, Ontario M2J 1P9, Canada
AUSTRALIA	Pergamon Press (Aust.) Pty. Ltd., P.O. Box 544, Potts Point, N.S.W. 2011, Australia
FRANCE	Pergamon Press SARL, 24 rue des Ecoles, 75240 Paris, Cedex 05, France
FEDERAL REPUBLIC OF GERMANY	Pergamon Press GmbH, Hammerweg 6, D-6242 Kronberg-Taunus, Federal Republic of Germany

First edition 1982
Reprinted 1982, 1983

Library of Congress Cataloging in Publication Data

Richards, B. A. (Brian Alfred) [Dick]
The topic of cancer.
Bibliography: p.
1. Cancer—Treatment. 2. Cancer—Philosophy
I. Title [DNLM: 1. Neoplasms. 2. Neoplasms—Therapy.
QZ 200 R514t]
RC270.8.R5   1981   616.99'406   81-15857

British Library Cataloguing in Publication Data

Richards, B. A. (Dick)
The topic of cancer
1. Cancer
I. Title
616.99'4   RC261
ISBN 0-08-025937-5

Printed in Great Britain by A. Wheaton & Co. Ltd., Exeter

DEDICATION

To those who work,
To those who fight back ignorance and confusion,
To those who raise their heads above the barricade,
To those who apply open minds,
And above all,
To those who need the help in their struggle against disease.

CONTENTS

INTRODUCTION

Men occasionally stumble over the Truth, but most pick themselves up and hurry off as if nothing had happened.

Winston Churchill

Nothing succeeds like success. And nothing fails like failure.

Considered in the broadest terms, orthodox cancer treatment today is a failure and a disgrace. Contemporary cancer management in a number of respects, constitutes professional malpraxis.

Consequently this book is part of an attempt to change the direction of the world's medical research. A monstrous task that is to be sure. But the effort must be made as we are all rushing headlong in the wrong direction.

For twenty years as a family physician in the same town in England, I carried out or supervised the orthodox medical cancer therapies I had been taught. They didn't really work. Speaking with the advantages of hindsight, it now seems remarkable that I never seriously questioned the methods just the same. Neither did any of my colleagues so far as I recall.

Time and again a patient I'd known for years got cancer, was operated upon and treated with radiation and drugs, and was returned to my care. The same routine then followed with remorseless repetition. I would begin the hopeless task of presiding over that patient's decline, telling reassuring lies, and giving more and more pain-relieving drugs until death ensued. What about those who got better? There were not enough to write about. Though so-called 'natural remissions' are said to occur, I was not lucky enough to have any actually come my way. My conclusion after a quarter of a century of medical practice is that truly spontaneous remissions from cancer are almost as rare as chicken's teeth. Indeed such cases as do occur are probably always the result of a re-instated bodily resistance that had been previously impaired. This is a theme to which this book will repeatedly return.

1

It took me shamefully long to realise that the methods we were all using were worthless failures. It then took several years more to find and learn better ways. But better ways do exist. This book is an attempt first to inform then to convince doctors, patients, and patients-to-be, of the existence and efficacy of these methods.

Unfortunately there is a snag. Everyone, doctors, research workers, and of course those prospective patients-to-be, the public, are conditioned to fear cancer, to regard its result as certainly fatal, and usually associated with great misery. Above all they regard modern unsuccessful treatments as depending utterly on surgery, radiation, anti-neoplastic drugs and on nothing else. The first of these concepts is wrong. The second is right.

Nevertheless these factors are all deeply ingrained into most people's overall view of cancer. To accept an alternative requires a paradigm shift of opinion; something very difficult to achieve.

If a researcher, working in a well recognised field, makes a small discovery, it is likely to be published in a learned journal. He has advanced a fragment of man's knowledge boundary by a tiny step into the still unknown. This worker will secure his just small acclaim and will incur no-one's wrath. However, let someone take an unexpected leap forward, perhaps in a field not entirely his own, and his action will tend to engender surprise, criticism, perhaps ostracism, and worst of all, lack of acceptance.

Yet we know that a vast proportion of the world's great advances have come about, not through painstaking research, but through brilliant innovation, vivid imagination, bold effort, and sheer fortunate accident.

Nowhere is this more true than in medicine. It is comfortable to stand still, quiet, undisturbed. There is a certain security in sheep-like lack of competition. Sheep are notoriously agitated by anything loud or moving. This may be part of the reason why the horrific results and inevitable failures of orthodox medicine are continually perpetrated without question, and why the rational and safe methods are rejected.

The medical press of the last year or two has contained numerous different opinions about cancer. Some groups of doctors have been experimenting (for that, at this stage, is what it amounts to), with the new exciting drugs that kill cancer cells. They have found that 'cocktails' of different drugs are more effective than the single drugs previously used. They are full of hope.

At the same time other specialists have pointed out that in real terms of cure, or substantially extended life span, some of the most prevalent cancers have shown no statistical improvement this century. That goes for both treatment and prevention of, for example, female breast cancer whether by surgery, irradiation, drugs, or mixtures of all three.

Things came somewhat to a well-publicised head when a British TV programme (Man Alive) revealed this little known fact. Such was the furor that further television time was devoted to discussion. At that time the Chairman of the Mastectomy Association (Betty Westgate) quite rightly pointed out that disclosure of the unfavourable facts must have disturbed many women. While she felt that the truth should be known, such blunt presentation might discourage women from seeking help.

With that entirely reasonable comment, she put her finger right on the point. Is it really help when the kind of treatment offered has been discredited?

The real truth is that the orthodox treatment of cancer of the breast in the year 1980 offers no significantly better chance of survival than it did in the year 1900. One series of tests after another has shown that whatever kind of operation is performed, with or without follow up irradiation, the expectancy remains obstinately unimproved. Though drugs are offering a very modest life extension, there is grave concern as to whether the kind of life experienced after treatment by the drugs is worth living at all.

Great hope was created by the arrival some years ago of regular breast screening. The intention was to find tumours in their early stages. The belief was that treatment in these earlier stages would be more successful. Gradually the accumulating statistics showed that life expectancy with breast cancer was at last beginning to increase. At least, that's what the figures seemed to show.

Now we know better. They show no such thing. What has happened is that the number of years a woman lives after discovery of a cancer is only longer because the cancer was found earlier. The woman dies at the same time, irrespective of treatment. It's just that, by then, more years have been counted. Only on paper has early detection appeared to extend the life span. Not only treatment but early detection has failed in this condition!

We must watch other early warning schemes with equal suspicion. There is the very real danger of pinning too much faith in them. What is more, people are inclined to make the error of thinking that early detection equates with prevention. It does not.

Orthodoxy in medicine has many benefits to patients. But it does tend to prove blinkered. Up to a century ago doctors accepted the association of cancer incidence with emotional states. As recently as 1950 famous surgeon Sir Heneage Ogilvie, noting the way cancers follow such disasters as bereavement, financial catastrophe or serious accidents, commented that "some controlling force that has hitherto *kept the outbreak in check has been removed*" (my italics).

Statistics are now available to show that cancer incidence *is* related to disasters of the type Ogilvie recognised. They show too that emotional states and personalities *do* influence the life expectancy in cancer. Discovery of the mind's ability to alter body function contributes to a new breadth of understanding. Recognition of external environmental factors like radiation and chemical pollution and cancer-encouraging agents is a further contribution. So is the increasing importance attached to the internal environment created by possibly injurious foodstuffs.

Boiling it all down to the bottom of the pot, one inescapable fact emerges. In cancer treatment, orthodoxy has failed and failed miserably, at astronomical cost in terms of both finance and human suffering.

As lawyer Ian Kennedy pointed out in the 1980 prestigious series of BBC Reith Lectures, the medical profession does not have a monopoly of potentially useful techniques. It is, of course, difficult for devoted and skilled physicians, who have dedicated years to orthodox cancer therapy, to recognise that it has all been a failure. It is natural for them to buoy themselves and their patients up with hopes of the impending breakthrough.

When orthodoxy fails it becomes the turn of unorthodoxy (perhaps heterodoxy is a better word). If doctors are too blinkered to make open-minded and objective judgements, then they forfeit the right to judge at all.

My own wish would be to see the undoubted skills of doctors turned to include alternative methods. I feel that these methods would be in safer hands, as would be the patients. I feel that the spectrum of abilities and understandings of the honoured physician and friend are invaluable and should be preserved. But only as long as there is no more conditioned scepticism or closed-minded rejection.

So called 'alternative' medicine has grown from three main sources. The 'old wives tales' embody much primitive but reliable folk memory, especially about diet, herbal remedies and health safeguards. Common sense, which is anything but common, inclines us away from cruel failures and towards more natural techniques. Finally, experience and observations are demonstrating that these methods do succeed.

As an interesting aside there is something that shows how opinion is steadily veering towards a change. In early 1978 I sent a serious article on the approaching trends of unorthodox cancer treatment to a major British doctors' publication, *World Medicine*, to which I had frequently contributed before. It was declined, as was the editor's privilege. This decision I accepted without comment and went on to contribute other things. But when I published a similar article for a more general readership in a non-medical publication, the Deputy Editor of *World Medicine* wrote and published a most offensive attack on me and my views.

I do not complain about that either. I mention it to demonstrate the view of established medical opinion in 1978. This year another major medical publication, *Doctor*, was pleased to accept and print my views.

A huge correspondence from doctors seeking further information ensued. And this year, too, no fewer than four prestige publishers were kind enough to compete for the manuscript of this book. That must mean something.

* * * * *

My standpoint, as author of this volume, is unequivocal. It is that cancer does not need to be treated with the wanton brutality now used. It must therefore stop. At once. There is an alternative way, better in many ways, painless, natural, thorough and at least equally successful. In contrast to current techniques of cut, burn and poison, it is truly a gentle method.

This book attempts to explain the Gentle Method and to show how and, above all, why, it should be adopted forthwith.

As we shall see, we are all getting cancer or potential cancer repeatedly as a more or less daily event. Yet, for the most part we overcome it virtually effortlessly. So, there are natural ways in which cancer can be, and is being overcome. In truth, did we but know it, and nearly all the time, cancer really is 'a beaten disease'.

* * * * *

May I conclude this introduction by acknowledging the work of others far greater than myself in this field. My own methods are, in large part, adopted and adapted from the pioneering efforts of others.

My thanks in abundance go to the many people who have helped me and contributed to this book, and to those whom I have quoted knowingly. My thanks too, perhaps even more so, to those teachers, writers, colleagues and patients who I have also quoted, probably without even realising the source of my thoughts.

CHAPTER ONE

THE TOPIC OF CANCER

The word cancer is now an unfortunate one. It has become accepted as if it were a word describing a certain disease. In fact, correctly used, cancer is a collective word for a whole series of diseases. There are probably in excess of two hundred and fifty kinds of cancer, most of them very rare. As the characteristics of different cancers vary so widely it is an oversimplification, perhaps, to classify them all together. However, some vital characteristics are held in common.

The best definition of cancer is that it consists of cells, growing at the expense of the organism in which they live and of which they are a part, but without serving any useful purpose in that organism. In effect, the cells form a group or mass, and go on growing, taking nourishment from the host, contributing nothing in return, and eventually causing serious danger to the host as a result of one or more factors.

Processes of cell and tissue growth under healthy conditions are by no means adequately understood. Some authorities consider that the natural state of healthy cells means continuous growth. As this would clearly not be in the interest of the entire organism, a series of control mechanisms have been developed and are in constant operation. When further cell growth is for any reason undesirable, the cells are spoken of as being repressed. They continue to live but there is no increase in the overall number of cells. Only enough new cells are produced to replace those succumbing to age or wear and tear. In other words the balance is maintained. Enough cells undergo division into two, in order exactly to balance cell wastage. The end result is that the overall number of cells remains roughly the same.

There are likely to occur episodes in any tissue, when there is a sudden need for more cells. For example, the skin may be injured, perhaps, in part removed. Immediately, the relevant cells are de-repressed. In the area concerned, and *only* in that area, cells begin to thrive, grow and proliferate in an effort to make up the damaged area. As the repair process nears completion there is gradually re-imposed the original methods of repression, now spoken of as re-repression. With the return of normal function, the earlier degree of cell growth and replacement is restored.

What can be seen from this simple example is that the degree of control is most precisely balanced. Cells may grow very rapidly indeed, as in the swiftly developing embryo. Or they may not increase in numbers at all, as is the case with nerve cells. But whatever rate of growth is in the genetically determined interest of the whole organism, then that rate is controlled by the delicate balance of repression and de-repression. Individual cells, as it were, have their interests subordinated to the interests of the whole.

In cancer, this control appears to be partially or wholly lost. The cancer cells grow and proliferate 'selfishly' in a way which sooner or later is very much contrary to the interest of the whole living creature.

There are several possible results of uncontrolled growth. The enlarging group of cells swells to form a mass more often known as a tumour. This tumour may bulge from the surface of the body in a way that is not only unsightly but additionally vulnerable to injury. Worse still, it may be an internal tumour, which on swelling, presses on other organs. This may cause pain or the impaired function of the compressed area. There may be resultant blockages. If hormone-producing cells become malignant, the increased numbers may result in a vast over-production of that hormone with consequent upsets of endocrine function.

Current orthodox medical opinion, which so far at any rate is correct, sees malignancy as an irreversible change of cell behaviour. It is thus deduced that the only things to do about malignant cells are either to remove or to kill them. As we shall later read, this deduction is not accepted by a growing number of doctors. Nevertheless, malignancy at present means that even when whatever stimulus it was that caused the cancer is ended or removed, the new growth (neoplasm) continues. Worse, luxuriant growth goes on at a headlong rate even when the host organism is at the point of extinction.

Before going into the causes of malignancy, it is as well to understand what exactly are the phenomena that characterise this destructive aberration of apparently normal functions. There are exceptions to the following list and not every cancer exhibits each characteristic. They do comprise a useful guide, however, and have been published as such by a leading textbook of pathology[1].

[1] Boyd, *Textbook of Pathology*, 1967.

First, on microscopic examination, it is immediately obvious that the nucleus of a malignant cell is different. It is larger in size in proportion to the cell containing it. It is also darker in colour, accepting more of the stains used to make cells easier to scrutinise under a microscope. When cells are in division (see Chapter 3) their nuclei adopt particular forms known as mitotic figures. Far more of these figures are seen in malignant tissues than in healthy ones.

There are many different kinds of cells in the body. Although they developed from one original fertilised egg-cell, over countless cell generations they have changed until, to the experienced eye, they can be easily differentiated one from another. This differentiation is lacking in malignant cells. Instead of looking like the presumed parent tissue cells, they come to resemble more primitive, perhaps embryonic-looking cells. This de-differentiation gives rise to one of the major theories of cancer causation to be discussed later.

Next, the cells tend to lose their customary neat or organised layout. This is called loss of polarity. Instead of cells being arranged, as is often the case, in neat rows, pallisades of similar sized cells, or layers and sheets, this orderly sequence is lost. Cells divide in what looks a haphazard way. Instead of ceasing to expand when they meet and touch neighbouring cells, as is the routine in health, malignant cells go on and on dividing, heaping up, piling over and into other cells in a totally uncontrolled manner.

Part of this cellular lack of concern for neighbouring territory results in the next characteristic, one of the most fearsome of all, that of infiltration. The madly proliferating cells squeeze against and between the healthy cells alongside them, whether they are part of the same organ or not. As a result, healthy areas are infiltrated by living strands of cancerous tissue probing out in many directions. It is probably from this infiltration that the word 'cancer' arises. For it derives from the Latin word for crab, as in the Zodiac sign Cancer; an allusion perhaps to the naked eye view of some cancers when sliced with a knife, and which then have vaguely radiating 'limbs' of tissue extending from a central zone.

Malignant tumours also appear to recur after removal. This may be a completely new tumour, caused by the same causes as produced an earlier growth. Often it is because some malignant tissue was missed at operation and survived to thrive again. Or some cells may have lain dormant in an unsuspected area. It may also be that malignant or pre-malignant cells exist far beyond the apparent boundaries of a tumour. Removal of the main centre does not prevent their eventual growth into fresh tumours.

Metastases is the name given to fragments of malignant tissue, similar to a main or primary tumour, but appearing as secondaries in other areas, often quite remote from the original. It is hypothesised that these are the result of single cells or small groups, separating from the primary tumour and being carried along in the bloodstream or lymphatic system. When they finally lodge somewhere, their growth produces another tumour.

The final characteristic of malignancy is that of progressive growth. Benign tumours eventually stop growing. In theory at least, malignant tumours do not. They are theoretically capable of going on growing until the host is destroyed. This raises an interesting possibility. Not all tumours do grow steadily, but may undergo slowed down periods. And as some tumours eventually cease to grow and are 'contained' or, as it were, fenced off from the surrounding body, these may be signs that the body is well able to defend itself against malignancy given the right circumstances. This is a very important theme, to which much attention will later be given.

"The condition of the environment may change and consequently damage the viability of [cancer] cells"[2]. For example the tumour tissue, like all other living tissues, depends upon blood supply for its needs of oxygen. If blood supply is cut, the tumour cells will die, or undergo necrosis. Also, extensive areas of fibrosis are often found around some old breast cancers. These represent areas of repair where the balance has been turned against the malignant cells.

This gives a great element of hope to the whole situation. Patients who have cancer do not usually die of it. Not directly. They die of the combination of weaknesses occasioned by the tumour. By the way it utilises vital supplies of nutrients. Or from the anguishing wear and tear of prolonged pain. From fear, from poisonous waste materials collecting in the body, or simply from wasting away when food intake can no longer equal bodily requirements. And some people die because of the wrong treatment.

Dr. Trevor Powles from a major British cancer hospital, The Royal Marsden, London, stirred up a hornet's nest quite recently when he suggested, in the hallowed pages of the *Lancet*, that far from improving survival in patients, modern chemotherapeutic (cytotoxic) drugs may actually reduce the life expectancy of some cancer patients.[3]

Other doctors, including two of his colleagues, wrote to dissociate themselves from the opinion. Nothing daunted, Powles retorted that claims of benefit from drugs may well be based more on enthusiasm than on fact. The violent disagreements and vehement proclamations of different 'experts' at cancer symposia are now well-known, as each defends his own pet programme.

If there is material in this chapter that sounds pessimistic, this

---

[2]*Ibid.*, p. 104.
[3]*General Practitioner*, May 16, 1980, p. 65.

latter kind of disagreement should give everyone renewed heart. Experts are disagreeing. Older horror-movie treatments are meeting more and more opposition. The trend is being set.

So we must get the whole concept of cancer into a new perspective. It is a prevalent condition. It is a dangerous condition. But although some twenty percent of people get it, the other eighty percent do not.

It is *not* inevitable that *you* will get it. And if you do, it is *not* inevitable that you will die. As we shall see, the chances of developing malignant disease can be vastly reduced. The chances of fighting it and overcoming it successfully can be enormously increased. For cancer can now be combatted both prophylactically and therapeutically by a whole campaign of new, sane, virtually non-toxic methods.

It is to that campaign that the huge sums devoted to cancer research should now be directed. Before dealing with that campaign, however, it is important to consider what are the causes of cancer, and why current concepts and therapies are so wrong and therefore so unsuccessful.

CHAPTER TWO

WHEN THE KILLING HAS TO STOP

I do know that in the overwhelming majority of cancers where a lot of money has been spent on diagnosis and therapy, neither the precocity of the diagnosis nor the kind of treatment used has any impact on the survival rates. We do have increasing evidence that those who are treated, supposedly for curative purposes, at best have an earlier onset of anguish, a prolonged period of impairment, and a greater intensity of pain than those who succeed in escaping the doctor.

Illich

*   *   *

I am left wondering why this good woman had to have her last weeks made a torment by . . . the wretched physical side effects of ineffectual drugs.

Gould

*   *   *   *   *

Cancer is one of the most common, vicious and swiftly increasing diseases in the world. Hundreds of thousands of otherwise healthy people will die of it this year. At least twenty per cent of humans born in Western society today will die of it. Millions of pounds, dollars, marks and francs have been spent on research into methods of cure in the last fifty years. Not only does the research and the money fail to stop cancer, it also fails to break even by curing as many new cases as occur annually. Indeed, it is worse than that. It fails even to retard the rate at which cancer increases momentum annually. Despite all the efforts, cancer gains rapidly in virtually every reliable set of newly published figures. The disease stubbornly resists all efforts to abate it.

13

At the present time, of the cancers that can be regarded as being of major significance, the commonest in women alone is breast cancer, and in men only, cancer of the lung. The commonest in both sexes together is cancer of the large bowel, the colon and rectum. All are horrific diseases.

The pattern has changed in the past and may change again in time. But current figures are alarming. Data collected by the USA National Cancer Institute and already published[1] demonstrate an overall and progressive increase of eleven per cent in the last forty years. More than twenty of the thirty-four types of cancer listed have increased, a third of them by more than seventy-five per cent. The same figures state that in the first half of the nineteen seventies, the increase was not merely in the well-known lung cancer and was thus not mainly due to smoking. Even when lung cancer is excluded from the calculations, the overall cancer increase for other areas of the body is hardly altered.

Each woman now has a greater than one in five chance of suffering an invasive malignant tumour some time in her life[2]. The age group in which cancer of the cervix of the uterus occurs is falling steadily. It is now not uncommon even in the twenties.

There is one seemingly bright feature in cervical cancer. Actual deaths from the disease have decreased overall[3]. Unfortunately they have increased in younger age groups. What is more, despite the huge expenditure on the cervical smear campaign, over two thousand women a year still die of the disease in the United Kingdom, even in well-screened populations. The campaign is clearly helpful but totally inadequate. However we look at the statistics, cancer remains rampant, prevalent and largely out of control, in spite of modern techniques of screening, supervision and treatment methods.

Could it be then, one might be forgiven for asking, that, after the miserable failure of present methods for so long, we might start to suspect that we are heading in the wrong direction? Statistics suggest that we are losing ground, not gaining it.

What is more, these unsuccessful methods are by no means harmless. Indeed, the very rationale behind them is that they should be dangerous, but more dangerous to the tumour cells than to the patient's remaining healthy cells. Surgery cuts the tumour out or off. It may then involve extensive dissection of the area and its lymphatic drainage network of lymph nodes to seek out possible disseminated secondaries spreading from the main growth. Surgery at this level is painful, carries a proportionate risk, and takes the patient a long time to recover,

[1] Epstein, Dr. S., *The Politics of Cancer*, quoted in *The Sciences*, Vol. 20, No. 7, Sept. 1980.

[2] Bromham, D. and Hull, M., Gynaecological cancer, *Journ. Mat. and Child Health*, Nov. 1980.

[3] Macgregor, J.E. and Teper, S., *Lancet*, 2 (7 Oct. 1978), 774-776.

meanwhile using up various bodily resources. Furthermore, even amongst doctors, there are grave doubts about the wisdom and the success of surgery.

Radiation of the affected zone by exposure to X rays and similar often follows surgery. The dose fatal to tumour cells is usually lower than that of healthy cells. But the difference is small and the appalling after effects of radiation sickness are described more fully in Chapter Four.

If the third stage of therapy is to be embarked upon, the seriously weakened patient now receives highly toxic anti-neoplastic drugs by mouth or by injection. This is the technique known generally as chemotherapy or treatment by chemicals, in this instance extremely poisonous ones. These aim to suppress the immune system, and kill off malignant cells. Their side effects are often profoundly unpleasant. It was such a case as this latter that is quoted by Dr. Gould at the head of this chapter.

There can be no doubt that all these 'cut, burn and poison' therapies would be justified in the vast majority of cases, as long as response was adequate and a cure resulted. However, not only, according to numerous patients, is the treatment worse by far than the disease itself, but it does not produce a cure . . . or anyway, not often enough.

While survival rates for cancer-like Hodgkin's disease are better now than they were, only about a fifth of leukaemias survive for five years. At the same time only six to eight per cent of lung cancers are alive at the five year mark[4]. In the United Kingdom, the numbers dying from breast cancer were 335 women per million in 1945, 350 in 1959, 383 in 1960, 426 in 1970, and 479 in 1979[5].

Success in orthodox therapy tends to be measured more or less statistically. It is the extension of the average anticipated life span that is the criterion. If a group of patients in a clinical trial of, say, a new anti-neoplastic drug, show a six week longer average survival time than a similar untreated 'control' group, then that new treatment is regarded as an advance in the anti-cancer regime. This surely is an instance in which every new set of figures should carry the Government Warning: Statistics can seriously damage your health.

For in them, no one considers the fact that the extra six weeks won for the patient are seldom weeks of health. They may well be six weeks of prolonged pain, profound weakness, emotionally stressful anticipation of death, nausea, vomiting and personally degrading loss of normal biolgical function. In other words, the life span is what is important. Left totally unconsidered is the quality of that extra few weeks of life.

---

[4] *Cancer Statistics: Survival.* H.M. Stationary Office.
[5] *Medical News*, 13 Nov. 1980, p. 4.

Yet, curiously, if you ask the average man in the street or the average doctor who works in cancer medicine, they will invariably agree that though life to them is sweet, it is really the quality of life that matters most and that they personally would not want to go on living if in pain, unhealthy, a burden to others and so on. They would prefer death to that kind of life.

Here, then, is an anomalous situation. Doctors and patients are striving to carry out treatments aimed in the very reverse direction to the principles they themselves purport to hold. This curious dichotomy stems from two social phenomena, both of which are related to the western hemisphere inhabitants' attitude to death.

There is a strange concept now widely held in our society that if anybody dies it must be someone's fault. In the medical professions particularly, this can take physical manifestations in the risks of litigation. It thus appears to the practitioner and to others, that it is vital to show that "everything had been done", that no medical technique that could have extended life has been untried, that death was the result of failure in an intense battle for life.

This is why we so frequently observe in the immediate pre-death period both patient and doctor acting out roles imposed on them by society, yet which both know to be mere worthless charades. Neither feels able to vacate the roles which have become accepted and which by their very performance, remove culpability from the participants. In fact, in the present climate of public opinion it is probably impossible for the physician not to issue unnecessary and even harmful drugs or to suggest ineffective surgical processes.

Another aspect, strange at first sight, has also been postulated. This is to suggest that many sufferers see cancer death as an acceptable form of suicide.[6] This comment is not restricted to those who have actually given up a painful and weary struggle, though it can be more obviously applied to them.

From personal observation it is possible to state, and to be repeatedly surprised that, an infinite majority of cancer sufferers do accept their fate. They may display much fortitude and courage, but it becomes quite clear that they have totally accepted their lot which they know involves a descent through unpleasant and unsuccessful therapies to an inevitable death. Their hopes revolve, not around the possibility of survival, but around not being a problem to others, remaining or being kept pain-free, and having an early, untroubled death. The general attitude can be summed up as a hope, associated with some personal effort, to enjoy the remaining timespan. What is conspicuously absent, usually, is any effort at all to extend that life span by aggressive means

---

[6] McNaughton, *A.R.L. Physicians Handbook of B17 Therapy*, Preface.

that embody genuine hope of survival.

Clearly, then, the stage which is set for the onslaught on or management of cancer cases, is deplorable. The despondent resignation of the entire cast to failure is matched only by paucity of the armamentarium and the blind persistence with unsuccessful methods of the past.

Another distasteful factor must be mentioned. I deliberately forbear to comment upon it and leave it to the individual to weigh its relevance. With a disease that currently kills perhaps six million human beings per year, there is an immense economic complex assembled around it. Combining those who work in research, treatment, administration, and all the associated supportive facilities, it is suggested that more people live off the proceeds of cancer than die from it. Thus, it is not possible to ignore a big business lobby in the corridors of power. There is no reason to assume that political and financial persuasions could not be active in this sphere as they have been in others.

Suspicion of this might be aroused by an event that recently occurred in the pages of a prominent international scientific publication[7]. In a book review a leading professor complimented an author for his criticism of professional medical inertia in failing to consider "alternative conception of the cause and care of cancer", in other words, innovative and alternative medicine techniques. This, he felt, was "intolerable in view of the relation between the shocking increase in the incidence . . . on the one hand and, on the other, the poisoning of the bio-sphere wrought by profit-hungry technology, most pointedly in the area of nutrition".

Another prominent doctor (Dr. C. H. Lushbough) protested in print that this kind of statement was less than responsible. In deliberate contradiction of published figures, he claimed that apart from smoking-related lung cancer, "all other major neoplastic disease (cancer) rates in the USA are either level or slowly declining".

One can only wonder whether his objection might not have carried more weight of honesty had Dr. Lushbough also stated that he is a board member of the American Cancer Society. The ACS line is widely held to be well accommodated to the corporate powers that control it. The line is roughly that, as cancer is not getting any worse, we needn't worry about new chemicals in our food. Dr. Lushbough is also a Vice-President of the Kraft Food Company!

There are plenty of possible causative factors for today's lamentable state of cancer therapy. Expansion of existing techniques like bigger and better cobalt radiation machines have produced only minimally better results. The professional establishment is traditionally immobile. The social attitudes are sterile. Commerce has much to lose. So, is the

---

[7]Kovel, Professor J., Einstein College of Medicine. *The Sciences*, Vol. 19, No. 9, *et seq.*

continuation of current stagnation inevitable?

It seems not. Already small but hopeful signs of change are detectable. For example, during the 1960's the dominant surgical opinion concerning cancer of the breast involved what is called radical mastectomy. Whereas local mastectomy means just the removal of the visible breast, the radical form of the operation includes removal of the muscles deep to the breast, right down to the rib cage. In addition the portion of the breast which extends up into the armpit, the axillary tail, is also exposed and removed, and the numerous chains of lymph glands in that region are extensively dissected out and removed. The operation is far longer, far more disfiguring, produces weakness of the arm on that side, as well as swelling due to impaired lymphatic drainage. Obviously it is also much more traumatic to the patient.

Rare and gallant was the surgeon who did not carry out this procedure on a proven breast malignancy. It was the only conceivable thing to do. Only very slowly has the idea changed. For it transpired that, yet again, the apparent and traditionally right thing to do was not the best thing. Now it is known[8] that patients with stage one or two malignancies do just as well with local removal and associated therapies. A small step perhaps, but one in the right direction and revealing that contemporary professional opinion is not always correct and can alter.

What is needed, though, is not a piecemeal change but a fundamentally different approach. I submit that the entire concept of cancer as currently held is wrong.

Take, for example, the opinion of the California Cancer Advisory Council, in whose publications[9] appears this statement:

> "In the evaluation of anti-tumour effect, only objective decrease in the size of measurable lesions . . . can be accepted as demonstrating anti-tumour effects by the compound under study. Subjective effects such as pain relief, increased appetite, weight gain, increased activities . . . are not evidence of anti-cancer effect."

Now, if by pursuing this principle the patient merely had to forego the alleviation of pain and the feeling of better health for a time in order to achieve a real and permanent cure, then that would be an excellent judgement. As there is no cure the excellence is highly questionable.

What has to be considered at this point is not just why twenty percent of people get cancer, but why the other eighty per cent do not. By regarding the tumour itself as the disease, a fundamental error is

---

[8] Fisher, B., quoted in *Doctor*, 20 Sept. 1979, p. 12.
[9] California Cancer Advisory Council (Report to), *Criteria for Response to Therapy*, p. 57.

made. For the tumour is not the disease, it is merely a symptom of the disease, as will be pointed out in Chapter Three.

Currently acceptable 'logic' does appear obvious when regarded in the following way. Something goes wrong so that a tiny cancer zone, or group of cells, appears somewhere in the body. Drawing on the body's supplies of oxygen and food to nourish it, it grows. Gradually it presses against or infiltrates into neighbouring tissues. It may spread to distant areas via the lymphatic or circulatory systems. Sooner or later a vital function is impaired or the tumour gets so big that the sufferer succumbs. There is every apparent reason to regard the tumour as the cause of all the trouble.

To fault the logic it is necessary to go a step further, earlier in the history, and ask why and how the tumour began in the first place and, having begun, how it was able to survive. These aspects of the problem are dealt with in far greater detail in Chapters Three and Four. The principle, however, can be stated now.

Cancer is a metabolic disease of the entire body. In such disordered conditions cancers are predisposed to, while natural combative processes are simultaneously curtailed. Only thus does the tumour form and thrive.

Put another way, we must start to regard cancer not as if it were some intruder, but as a normally healthy process gone wrong; as something tolerated within the unhealthy body and permitted to remain due to impaired corrective mechanisms. It is vital to comprehend this point.

Nature, or rather, the healthy living body, has a way of coping with almost every problem, every disease, every infection. With the exception of trauma so sudden or so severe as to interrupt essential living processes, physiological mechanisms exist which can and do combat all kinds of ill-health. Cancer is not an exception to this rule.

Long before the arrival of antibiotics the overwhelming proportion of human infections were nevertheless combatted successfully. It usually took longer but there was a compensating bonus in that there was likely to be a greater degree of longer lasting immunity. A broken bone will heal, not always in the best functional position perhaps, but sufficiently to permit a return to a degree of function. This was so even before the discovery of immobilisation or plaster of Paris. Foreign bodies embedded in skin or muscle may be ejected as part of the contents of a boil formed around it. Conversely they may be effectively sealed off and contained, still within the body, but affording no serious threat.

Cancer, too, can be successfully combatted. Indeed, according to some eminent workers and thinkers[10] it is being so combatted, in all of us, as a daily occurrence. Minute tumours are detected by the immune

[10]Macfarlane-Burnett, Sir. *The Endurance of Life.*

system when comprised of a single cell or few cells. Recognised as aberrant cells, as 'non-self', these cancerous cells are treated differently from cells of the kind recognised as belonging to 'self'. They are differently treated by exposure to specially and swiftly manufactured antibodies and by specialised white blood cells, lymphocytes.

As long as the defence mechanisms are intact successful elimination of the potential growth is accomplished. Unfortunately, the very conditions which predispose to tumour formation also limit effective natural responses.

Malignant disease must be regarded as an accident of nature, which, like other accidents of nature, can be cured. The aim must be to aid the normal processes of resistance to, and attack on, malignant tissues. In this overall plan it is a mistake to regard the problem as entirely physical.

While physicians are growing more and more conscious of the psychosomatic aspects of disease and the growing number of emotional disorders presenting with physical symptoms, they have a curious reluctance to accept the relevance of the psyche in something as physical as malignancy. It is wrong to draw such a distinction.

Willpower or mere attitude of mind may not speed the union of a broken bone but it can certainly hasten the progress to the point where the limb is in full healthy function again. It has no less importance to cancer. I have seen repeatedly how psychic amplification of negative factors like fear, remorse, and self-pity militate against a patient, whereas concentration on positive factors like determination, love and resistance are immensely beneficial. Because the psychic effects cannot be reproduced or measured in laboratory animals is no reason to ignore their profound importance in man. In general, quitters succumb, fighters survive.

It could be assumed, then, that there is at least a case for a reappraisal of our views on cancer in general and in our methods of preventing and treating it in particular. If currently held theories are proving untenable and if contemporary therapeutic measures are continuing to fail, it is at least arguable that it might be time to abandon them in favour of more successful ways.

Yet that is not happening. Although the medical professions should naturally be anxious to advance cancer therapy, it does not appear that way. In spite of admitted awareness of their methods' limitations they continue to use and recommend them. They appear ignorant of nutritional and naturalistic therapies to the point of denying their efficacy without knowledge or experience. The few who try them, doctors and nurses alike, are swiftly converted. Those who will not try, even to learn with an open mind, actively discourage their patients from seeking any but the pathetic methods already on offer and almost guaranteed to be without success.

It is this constant repetition of failure that is proving so daunting to a small but growing number of people. Doctors in general *know* their methods are appallingly painful and that they have a near total lack of success. Yet they go on and on using them. This is the kind of tactics that prompted the quotations at the start of this chapter.

Ivan Illich is a world famous author and thinker, especially on medical matters. His works[11] have been read by hundreds of thousands. Yet he feels that cancer sufferers are better off when they are left untreated than when they receive the entire benefits of modern medical science!

Dr. Donald Gould, on the other hand, is an English family physician noted for the good sense of his commentaries and for his warmth and humour. After one of his friends had been treated unsuccessfully with debilitating chemotherapeutic drugs to within a few days of her wretched death, he felt obliged to ask his question in print.[12]

These gentlemen are in good company. Nobel Laureate, Sir MacFarlane Burnett expressed his opinion[13] that the sum total of satisfying life would probably be increased if, when a condition is recognised that has less than a 50% chance of definitive cure, treatment should be limited to what is necessary to offer comfort, irrespective of its effect on length of survival. This would most certainly exclude nearly all contemporary orthodox methods of treating malignant disease! Interestingly enough, it would not exclude the newer better methods this book proposes.

Gradually more and more people are feeling and expressing doubts. Are we justified in going on with these atrocious measures knowing the success is minute? Should we not be searching now for entirely new methods that might emulate natural and successful anti-neoplastic measures?

Such methods do exist. They are, by comparison, inexpensive, simple, and pain free. They have far fewer side-effects; they make the patient feel better and happier. And they work successfully against cancer. Assembled together, they comprise the Gentle Method.

Some of the comments in this chapter may, at first sight, appear too depressing, even demoralising. The problem at the moment is glum indeed. But there is this to be said to cancer sufferers and sufferers-to-be. Although orthodoxy has failed, and although the present state of therapy is deplorable, the newer, better, alternative methods are here and are gaining ground all the time.

So no-one should lose heart. Everyone should campaign. And every

---

[11] Illich, Ivan, *Medical Nemesis.*

[12] Gould, Dr. D., Comment, *General Practitioner*, 28 Sept. 1979, p. 37.

[13] As 10.

individual should fight to prevent and, if necessary, to overcome cancer. There must be no question of giving up. After all, look what you might miss if you die too soon!

Everyone must fight for life. And the fight *must* go on.

CHAPTER THREE

CANCER AND ITS CAUSES

Cancer is always the result of a fault developing in a natural healthy function. In other words, some perfectly normal living process, which previously worked satisfactorily, undergoes a change, the result of which is no longer health but disease.

The fault that develops is either a part of, or something that closely affects the normal sequence of cell division or mitosis. Mitosis is the process by which growth of the body takes place. Consider a single cell. It consists of three main parts. The main bulk of the cell, made up of living material, largely protein, is called the cytoplasm. The cell is surrounded by a limiting layer that forms its boundary, the cell membrane. It is through this that all materials must enter or leave the cell, and it is on this membrane that many external substances effect their influence upon the cell. Finally, there is a darker, more dense area, often towards the centre of the cell, called the cell nucleus.

Part of the content of the nucleus is the material chromatin, much of which is comprised of the complex proteins that form the chromosomes. Chromosomes are straight or slightly curved rod-shaped structures of exact number and content in each living creature. Highly magnified they are found to consist of a series of smaller fragments, the genes. These are the protein molecules that carry coded information about the tissue, what it is, how it should grow, its shape, size and so on. The major component is deoxyribonucleic acid or DNA.

It is the arrangement of different protein precursors, amino-acids, forming the DNA molecule that carries the essential coding for every characteristic about any specific plant or animal. By their sequence they carry a code that is passed on from each cell generation to the next. Not only obvious factors like size, shape and colour are so coded. Down to the minutest detail everything is coded. The rate at which individual

23

cells are to develop, in which direction, how far, are programmed side by side with the kind of enzymes and chemical reactions that will take place in the cell.

Some idea of the complexity of the human genetic code can be imagined from the estimate[1] that it would require a thousand books, each of two thousand pages, to describe a single human cell. Yet the DNA content of that single cell, if stretched out on a desk-top, would be only a little more than six feet long.

DNA has another remarkable ability, that of replication. It is replication that is responsible for passing on the information store to the next cell in line. Described in general terms the process is as follows. When a cell has grown to a certain size, or when some other stimulus indicates the need, the sequence of events of mitosis begins. First, the nucleus becomes even more than usually dark in shade. Then the chromosomes become more distinct and easily seen.

At this stage the vital process of replication takes place. Each fragment of DNA in turn attracts towards it complementary chemical fragments from the contents of the cell. These new amino-acids are lined up along the original DNA molecule until an exact copy has been made. It is the exactness of this process that allows use of the word, replicate. For the result is an identical copy of the original DNA.

Replication is far from the simple and automatic pairing up of nucleotides that once was pictured. One method involves the unwinding of short segments (Okasaki pieces) of DNA in which an "unwinding enzyme" is involved. At the end of each segment an opening is made and a short sequence of ribonucleic acid (RNA) is inserted as an initiator for the replication process. This requires an elaborate set of enzymes programmed in a way that is not yet understood, to locate the right place and insert the correct number and sequence of ribonucleotide molecules. Another complex process then takes place in which the new strand is progressively lengthened, nucleotide by nucleotide, each being paired with the complementary nucleotides on the pattern of the template strand. At each stage a number of different enzymes must recognise from the template which nucleotide is required, extract it from the cellular pool of supplies (which must be constantly replenished), and insert it in the exact position. As the segment is completed, other enzymes then remove the temporary RNA primer, rejoin the segment to the completed part of the new DNA molecule, and ensure that the two strands twist around each other to form the correct and familiar double helix.

When all the gene material has been precisely copied, the two new sets of material, parent and offspring, draw apart so that there is a gap

[1] Rich, Professor A., Biophysics Dept., Massachusetts Institute of Technology.

between them in the cell. Briefly, the cell has two entire sets of nucleus material in two separate nuclei. The cytoplasm now divides down between the nuclei so that two new cells are formed, the new generation cells each containing an entire set of coded genetic information.

Clearly the replication has to be utterly exact. This is how skin cells form new skin, and liver cells form new liver, not vice versa. But nothing even in Nature is entirely perfect, all of the time. Errors do occur. The process of replication, though appearing simple under a microscope, is, in reality, anything but. Numerous other chemicals are used to assist what is a most complex mechanism.

When errors do take place other enzymes take over and attempt to repair the fault. As is obvious from the way creatures do live and grow 'properly' most of the replication and its repair processes work satisfactorily. But even after all the detailed activities have been completed, errors do occur and fail to get corrected.

The snag is that once an error has escaped correction it may well become embodied into the genetic code. When the time comes for the next cell division, the error will be copied along with the correct material. It is perpetuated into forthcoming cell generations. This is a potential source of great danger.

One of the vital constituents of the genetic code is that which will govern the rate of growth and division of the cells concerned. Cells cannot be permitted to grow on and on or to divide to form more every time they are big enough. Such a growth under optimum conditions would be at a colossal rate, spoken of as exponential. Living and dividing this way, a single celled creature, say one lone bacterium, would produce a kilogram of bacteria at the end of twenty-four hours, and a million million metric tons of it in a further twenty-four![2] The need for control is clear enough.

When malignancy occurs, and that control is lost, it is probably always due to a fault arising in the genetic DNA coding. The result may be a cell that grows exceedingly fast, resulting in a cancer of high malignancy. If the rate is slower, the cancer is of low malignancy. The conditions under which the cancer grows are never the optimum mentioned in the bacteria example above. There are other restraining and resisting influences that restrict the innate malignancy rate of the tumour.

If a tumour, started from an individual malignant cell, grows by regular division, it would need thirty divisions or doublings to form a mass one centimetre across[3]. At low malignancy rate of one doubling per hundred days, this would take eight to ten years to achieve a fist-

---

[2] Macfarlane Burnett, *The Endurance of Life.*
[3] Illingworth and Dick, *Textbook of Surgical Pathology*, 1979, p. 40.

sized mass. Moderate malignancy, doubling every thirty days, would take two or three years. High malignancy, which effects doubling at about ten day intervals, would require only one year.

*   *   *   *   *

Clues about the causes of cancer can even be found from the recorded medical history of the disease. The first known mention was in an Indian manuscript, the Ramayana, dating from about 2000 BC. This mentions cancer treatment not only by the knife (surgery) but by arsenic compounds, a kind of primitive chemotherapy. An Egyptian papyrus from 1500 BC also shows that they knew of different kinds of tumours, perhaps of different cause, and requiring different treatment.

Hippocrates, who is believed to have lived from 460 to 375 BC, divided tumours into innocuous and dangerous, or as we now classify them, probably similarly, benign and malignant. He it was who coined the word Karkinoma (from the Greek word *karkinos* = crab) which, as carcinoma, is still used to describe one large group of malignant conditions.

But it was the physician Galen (AD 131-201) who grouped tumours as being of three types. There were those which were 'according to Nature', such swellings as the abdomen after food, the joints if injured and, of course, the swelling of pregnancy. Then there were those that exceeded Nature, the natural swellings that sometimes became too great, like excess callus formation around broken bones. Finally there were tumours that were 'contrary to Nature', the whole series of benign or malignant growths.

Cancer, mass, tumour, swelling, neoplasm, carcinoma or growth, irrespective of its name it is the question of malignancy that matters most; that and its degree. What, then, causes this aberration of normal programmed function into headlong, uncontrolled and invasive growth?

Several causes are well known. Indeed it has been difficult in the last few years to find a time when there has not been argument over some substance or other alleged to be cancer-causing or carcinogenic.

In older times it was known that sweeps and others working with soot developed cancers in the scrotal region, believed to be the result of the soot-contained chemicals being rubbed into the unwashed skin for years on end. Other chemicals are now known causes. In fact, almost any substance applied excessively or for too long to an area seems able to bring about malignant change.

It is not so much value, then, to know merely what can cause cancer, as that includes practically everything. The important thing is also to discover *how* cancer is caused. There are three major theories, that cancer can be inherited, exogenous in that it is caused by external factors acting on the body, or endogenous in that internal factors are responsible.

Hereditary factors are undoubtedly relevant. Although conclusive evidence is lacking, every doctor can recount instances where cancer, often the identical kind of cancer, crops up repeatedly in members of the same family. A classical example of this was the family of the Emperor Napoleon. He is believed by most to have died of stomach cancer. So did his sisters, his father and his grandfather[4]. Quite certainly, too, some human cancers like retinoblastoma, an eye tumour of children, are inherited. This involves embryonic cells from which the retina develops.

Racial factors are also relevant, though these may be associated too with the usual geographical location of the race. Racial equality appears to have no adherents where such things are decided. For example, some Far Eastern peoples have low rates of stomach cancer. If they move to other areas, the rate increases to similar rates found in that area's indigenous population. One may wonder whether dietary or other environmental factors may not therefore be significant.

More cancers occur, of many types, in later age groups. While some tumours are restricted to the very young, these are comparatively uncommon. Most of the common cancers obey the basic rule. It may be that DNA errors accumulate to an unacceptable degree. Certainly cancer and age have many associations. These will be mentioned again in Chapter Seven, when the advantages of Regenerative Therapy are discussed.

Some cancers undoubtedly occur more in one sex than the other. In part this is a matter of the different organs of the two sexes. Cancer of the uterine cervix can exist only in the female, and of the penis only in the male. But other cancers in areas which are not obviously sex related also show different occurrence rates in males and females. The influence of sex hormones may well be the reason for some of these.

Some physical diseases are closely connected with the immune system. This is the process by which the body resists infections. If there is excessive activity of the system it may not only attack invading bacteria but parts of the body too. This is what happens in arthritis. There is some evidence that immunological factors can cause malignant growth. One example is cancer of the cervix in women of promiscuous habits. Cervical cancers caused through this are thought to be due to reaction against different kinds and contents of male semen. It is largely restricted to very young women in whom the cervix was still in, or only just emerging from, the period of very active growth of the area that comes with sexual maturity.

[4] Anderson and Kissane, Vol. 1, p. 670.

Extrinsic factors are notorious carcinogens. The erstwhile accepted association of physical damage with female breast cancer has been discredited. It is still believed, though, that trauma is associated with bone and muscle tumours arising in young people. Continuous or repeated friction of an area, as in nervous habits like picking or scratching, may give rise to new growth. Some apparently inert materials like polythene, if embedded in the skin, can also initiate malignancy.

So, without doubt, can radiation. This need not be in the form of radioactive fallout, though such a danger is sure enough. The medical use of radiation is also a cause of vast amounts of exposure. Ultraviolet light is another offender well known to cause skin cancers on those who are repeatedly exposed to it. Another factor causing increasing concern is the prolonged exposure to radar, microwave emission, television and electronic (digital) equipment sources.

Many chemicals can cause cancer. These include the soot already mentioned, mineral oils, tar, and of course cigarette smoke. Arsenic, cadmium, chromium, vinyls, carbon tetrachloride and food additives, like butter yellow, have all been conclusively implicated. So have some of the drugs used in cancer therapy (!) like nitrogen mustard, actinomycin and cyclophosphamide.

Biological offenders like viruses, substances that exist somewhere on the border line between living creatures and chemicals, are known cancer causers.

Emotional factors can also be implicated. Ogilvie's opinion (see Introduction) of the effect of bereavement is only one of many such significant comments.

One major cancer theory that enjoyed a brief vogue before falling into surprising neglect, is now gaining credibility again. This is known as the trophoblast theory. This was first suggested by the Edinburgh zoologist and embryologist John Beard (1857-1924). In essence, the theory suggests that embryonic material may survive in the adult and be activated, or perhaps de-repressed, at a later stage to initiate a malignant growth. Quite certainly the many similarities between cancer cells and trophoblasts are striking and have been well studied in the past[5]. However, it has also been pointed out[6] that when embryonic tissues are surgically transplanted into a host, they do not change their character. Instead of showing malignant tendency, they behave exactly as they should.

Some factors nevertheless appear suspicious. The endocrine profile, a tabulated series of estimates of circulating hormones, has shown the presence of embryonic hormones like chorionic gonadotrophin (HCG),

[5] Gurchot, C., *Biology: Key to the Riddle of Cancer*, 1949, p. 336.
[6] Oberling, C., *The Riddle of Cancer*, pp. 26-27, Yale University Press, 1946.

adrenocorticotrophic hormone (ACTH) and thyroid stimulating hormone (HCT), in a wide variety of cancer cases.

In the absence of certainty, an abundance of theories of the possible causes of cancer is inevitable. At one point, however, all theories converge. All are agreed that there is a point between cancer and non-cancer. There is a dividing line, or perhaps a dividing phenomenon. Before that takes place, the cell or tissue may be regarded as normal or, at most, pre-malignant. After that point the cell is quite certainly malignant.

It is at this precise point that the cause, or perhaps one should now say, the result, is understood. The cell has changed from a normal to a malignant state. Or, far more likely, a malignant cell has arisen from a non-malignant one. In effect, the new cell is no longer an exact replica of its parent. A change has occurred in the DNA that has altered the cell in one or more of its vital characteristics.

The new cell starts to exhibit some or all of the qualities of malignancy listed previously. We are left therefore with only two possible explanations. Either a potentially malignant cell, perhaps of the embryonic or trophoblast type, has always been present and has become suddenly de-repressed, or a cell has undergone a form of mutation from its original condition. When a cell mutates the resulting mutant may be deficient in some vital way. If so, it succumbs. Alternatively the mutant form may be capable of survival but is destroyed by other body processes soon to be discussed. Finally, the third possibility is that the new cell has, because of its changes, acquired not deficiencies but advantages. If those advantages are such that they enable it to grow, divide and thrive at the expense of other cells, out of proportion to need, and while maintaining an ability to avoid destruction by protection mechanisms, a "successful" tumour begins to develop. Cancer has started.

Mutation, then, can occur spontaneously as a result of DNA replication error. This is endogenous or intrinsic mutation. Mutation can also occur as a result of external influences like chemicals or radiation. Either way, if DNA repair fails, the mutant cell is poised to start growth.

That a single cell is usually, if not always, responsible for initiating a tumour is now a widely held view[7]. Many tumours and leukaemias have been thoroughly investigated and found to be monoclonal, and therefore derived from such a single mutant cell.

Nobel prizewinner Sir Macfarlane Burnett, probably the most brilliant and visionary biologist and embryologist of the last two generations, has expressed the opinion that something like one cell

---

[7]Fialkow: The use of genetic markers to study cellular origin and development of tumours in human females, *Advanced Cancer Research*, 15, pp. 191-226, 1972.

division in every million produces a potentially malignant mutant cell. As countless millions of cell divisions are constantly taking place, this means that everyone gets cancer, or at least the start of it, as often as several times a day.

The extreme complexity of replication and mitosis has already been explained. Complex processes are prone to greater error than simple ones. It should thus come as no shock that replication errors are common, and that malignant mutants occur with such frequency.

What appears more surprising is that serious disease results so rarely. One 'tissue' in the body in which it is comparatively easy to count cells, is blood. At a fair estimate each pint might contain two and a half million million cells. Most solid tissues are of far higher cell density. A wild estimate of the number of cells in the body can thus be made. Estimating the turnover of cells as once every hundred days, one might easily arrive at a guessed figure of three million million cell divisions a day. The true figure is probably substantially higher.

Irrespective of the detail of accuracy, what is sure is that perhaps several million potential malignancies occur in the average twelve stone man (168 lb, or 76 kg) each day. Yet in seventy years of life there is only a one in five chance that just one single one of those potential millions of malignancies becomes active cancerous growth. It is obvious that some very efficient protective mechanism is at work, if only that miniature proportion of malignant cells manage to survive.

This is the 'controlling force' that Sir Heneage Ogilvie suspected to exist. In fact these aberrant cells are located and eliminated by the function of the immune system so thoroughly that we are never aware of their existence. The most impressive evidence of this comes from the way in which malignancies occur so frequently in patients whose immune response is suppressed by drugs or in children born with deficient immune system function.

A constant surveillance system operates. Malignant cells do not belong where they are. Their characteristics are sufficiently different for them to be recognisable to the immune system as being 'non-self'. Once recognised they are attacked both by white blood cells (lymphocytes) and by chemical agents. It is likely that these latter are similar to the agents used to attack other intruding bodies such as bacteria.

Foreign material entering the body is known as an antigen. If it is potentially dangerous, the immune system manufactures chemicals called antibodies. These are individually made so that they can attach to and neutralise the antigen, thus rendering it harmless. (It is antibodies 'manufactured' by host animals against some infectious bacteria that are injected into humans in the process of immunisation.) Not only does the immune system produce an immense variety of antibodies. It has some kind of 'memory' system. It is only necessary for the same antigen to enter the body again, perhaps after an interval of years, for fresh anti-bodies to be produced often within a matter of a few minutes.

It is now possible to summarise the position in one sentence. Either from re-depressed embryonic cells reactivating, or from somatic muta-genesis, malignant 'seed' cells form which are then attacked and usually eliminated by vigilant defence mechanisms.

This search and destroy surveillance succeeds almost all of the time. As such it is of interest, but not of primary interest here. What matters more is why and how it fails on the rare occasions when it does.

Clearly the correct functioning of any bodily process must depend on an adequate state of health. The entire body must be healthy. The body does not consist, as many of us were inclined to be taught, of a series of different, separate systems. It is not like a house in which there is a hot water system, an electrical system, a ventilation system and so on. The digestive system, respiratory system, nervous system and other systems of the body are not simply grouped together within the same unit, merely as separately functioning systems. Rather the contrary; each and every part of the body exists in a state of inter-dependence with everything else.

It is illogical to treat one isolated part in most instances. It is the whole organism that is ill, even if the resulting symptom is only apparent at one particular spot. So, when a person gets cancer, it is because the whole person is ill, or ill-functioning. The defence mechanisms have broken down. Surveillance has failed. Cancer gets the upper hand.

This raises another new problem. Having considered the numerous internal and external influences that can cause cancer, we must devote at least equal importance to what factors can or may permit the new-born cancer to survive. What things are able so to limit, or thwart, the seek and destroy capability of the body's usually victorious defences.

For there are now seen to be not one but three possible ways of tackling the cancer problem. Most people know of the cut, burn and poison methods of orthodox therapy. A growing number are also starting to comprehend the value of reducing possible carcinogenic features in the environment. A smaller, but also growing number, are realising that a third method exists, that of promoting the counter-attack potential of anti-cancer defensive measures aimed at cure of the already created tumour.

This latter is an entirely new concept to most people, including those in the medical profession. Combined with an aggressive prophylactic routine, hitherto held by most to be impossible, the entire anti-cancer campaign is at last achieving a new recognition. It becomes more and more apparent that there really are measures that can prevent cancer, cure it when it occurs, or at the very least, largely reduce the numbers of cancers that develop to danger level.

*   *   *   *   *

A feature associated with cancer and which of late years has been puzzlingly neglected, is stress. This may operate as a cause of cancer, though evidence for this is so far lacking. What seems more logical is that the effect of stress is felt more at a level of defensive system curtailment.

Undoubtedly excessive stresses and strains do put pressure on available resources in a number of ways. Theories have been put forward that anti-stress responses utilise dietary components, vitamins or minerals, that are in short supply. Others think the mechanism may be one of the under- or over-production of adrenal hormones. Endorphins, chemicals produced in the central nervous system in reaction to pain, or other similar, as yet undiscovered, substances may also play a part.

A possible mechanism for the effect of stress has been suggested[8]. In experiments in the National Cancer Institute, Maryland, USA, laboratory mice were deliberately stressed by being kept immobilised in plastic tubes for eighteen hour periods. After this stress it was noted that white blood cells, normally active in attacking tumour cells, had undergone a 76% reduction in their efficiency at the task, even when stimulated by immunopotentiators such as interferon. The scientists also found that hormones from the adrenal glands (cortisone-type) which undergo much increase in production in stress situations, had a suppressant effect on the white cells. Their conclusion was that the stress-induced hormone rise was at least partly responsible for the impaired cell function. This creates a problem in that similar hormones (steroids) are widely used in orthodox cancer therapies. Yet another reason why the use of orthodox methods may be misguided and in need of revision.

Whatever the mechanism, one thing is very important. It is not only the stressful event that is significant. It is the quality of change that it brings about in the bodily routine that is at least equally important. Otherwise expressed, it is not merely the loss of the spouse and the associated grief that is relevant; it is the change in circumstances that results. Because of this even the loss of a hated spouse is an important stress factor. Furthermore, the common advice given to someone to have a change, or to change homes or jobs, may well be the worst possible thing.

Two workers, Holmes and Rahe, have produced a social readjustment scale attempting to relate various stressful incidents to the major stress of spouse loss. It is reproduced below (page 33) with the reminder that it is intended as a guide only, and one with possible wide

[8]Pavlides, N. and Chirigos, M., *Psychosomatic Medicine*, 1980, Vol. 42, No. 1.

Life event	*Mean stress value*
Death of spouse	100
Divorce	73
Marital separation	65
Jail term	63
Death of close family member	63
Personal injury or illness	53
Marriage	50
Fired at work	47
Marital reconciliation	45
Retirement	45
Change in health of family member	44
Pregnancy	40
Sex difficulties	39
Gain of new family member	39
Business readjustment	39
Change in financial state	38
Death of a close friend	37
Change to different line of work	36
Change in number of arguments with spouse	35
Mortgage over £10,000	31
Foreclosure of mortgage or loan	30
Change in responsibilities at work	29
Son or daughter leaving home	29
Trouble with in-laws	29
Outstanding personal achievement	28
Wife begins or stops work	26
Begin or end school	26
Change in living conditions	25
Revision of personal habits	24
Trouble with boss	23
Change in work hours or conditions	20
Change in residence	20
Change in schools	20
Change in recreation	19
Change in church activities	19
Change in social activities	18
Mortgage or loan less than £10,000	17
Change in sleeping habits	16
Change in number of family get-togethers	15
Change in eating habits	15
Vacation	13
Christmas	12
Minor violations of the law	11

personal variations. It will be noted that even things normally regarded as pleasant or happy can have prominent stress associations. For example, marital reconciliations, Christmas and holidays. A notable omission is the effect of deliberately stressing activities like competitive sports, strenuous exercise, sexual encounters or exciting spectacular occupations like watching games with emotional associations, horror movies, and so on.

It has long been propounded that there is a 'cancer-type' of person[9]. The suggestion is that he or she is the unfortunate sort of person, never thriving, enjoying mediocre health, vulnerable to stresses, accident prone, seldom successful. This group of characteristics may be the result of a low 'life-force' quotient in the sense of a congenital lack of drive and initiative. Or it may be induced by dietary deficiencies. The axiom that happy people don't get cancer may not be strictly true, but I personally find there is a lot in it. The fulfilled, involved, mildly hypertensive, sexually active extrovert who has an abundance of enthusiasm, features far less often on the lists of cancer diagnosis than those who are shy, nervous, discontented, vegetarian, low-sexed and restrained of habit.

An important piece of research reported in the leading British medical publication, *The Lancet*, in 1979[10], dealt with the different responses of women to the diagnosis of breast cancer. Cases were categorised as one of four possible groups. The first group was composed of those who denied the diagnosis. They declined to accept that they had cancer at all. Even if they underwent mastectomy, they would claim that it was only as a precautionary or preventative measure. The second group were those showing an aggressive fighting spirit. They sought to attack, fight and beat the disease in every way available. Third were those of stoic acceptance. They were perhaps distressed to start with, but as the anguish was overcome they determined to carry on with life as well and as long as possible. Finally there were those who were utterly overwhelmed by the diagnosis and who reacted only with helplessness and hopelessness.

These four groups were monitored for five years. The comparative figures are interesting:

	Group 1	Group 2	Group 3	Group 4
Percentage alive at 5 years with no recurrence	70%	80%	37%	20%
Percentage dead	10%	10%	29%	80%

[9]Cutler, Max, *Psychological Variables in Human Cancer*, 1954, p. 11.
[10]Greers, S., Morris, T., Pettingale, K.W., Kings College Hospital. *Lancet*, 13.10.79, 2, 785-7.

It cannot be deduced from these remarkable figures that it was emotional response alone that was relevant. For example, more members of the first two groups may have sought further information and, as a result, more successful therapies, like the Gentle Method described in the last sections of this volume. Nevertheless it is reasonable to conclude that whatever other factors are operating, strongly positive methods of interference, active combatting of the disease, encouragement of powerfully motivated and, hopefully, clinically effective emotional counter-attacks, must be regarded as prominent features of cancer management.

Dr. H. Nieper, one of the most eminent and successful of specialists in cancer therapy, has said[11] that he regards as a major problem the ability of malignant cells to shield themselves against immune system attack, by virtue of a mucoid layer that surrounds them much in the way found in some embryonic tissues. This may result from the possibly trophoblastic origin. He further feels that the shield depends, at least in part, upon electro-magnetic phenomena. Whatever the features of the shield, de-shielding is essential before the enclosed malignant cells can be attacked.

Nieper feels that the shield can be breached with the use of enzymes like Bromelains and vitamins, especially vitamin A or similar compounds of the beta-carotene type. He is also convinced of the embryonic origin of cancers. As evidence he quotes that tumour cells from mice, if cloned, that is, if allowed to develop to their maximum, produce new mice which are entirely normal. The initiating cell therefore must have been genetically malignant or pre-malignant, he claims.

Another widely acclaimed physician, Dr. E. Contreras, attempted to summarise the relevant factors of cancer aetiology and protection which might act on any given individual[12] (see the table on page 36).

*   *   *   *   *

In conclusion it must be said that the whole story of the aetiology of cancer is far from known. New carcinogens are constantly being discovered. The important facts are less what the small individual causes are, than what are the main groups of causes, how do they act, and how can they be combatted.

The main values of the discussion of cancer causation in this chapter are intended to be the ventilation of neglected but important theories, and the acceptance of the multiplicity of possible factors. From these are developed many of the preventative and therapeutic measures which comprise the Gentle Method.

[11] Lecture at Royal Society of Medicine, London, May 1980.
[12] *Ibid.*

Factors working for the patient	*v*	*Factors working against the patient*
Body anti-tumour mechanisms (white cells, antibodies, etc.)		Carcinogens (chemicals, radiation, (smoking, etc.)
Adequate nutrition		Poor nutrition (low minerals, junk foods, etc.)
Anti-tumour supplements (Selenium, zinc, etc.)		Shock from non-related surgery, disease, etc.
Medical therapies (unorthodox) (enzymes, amygdalin, mega-vitamins, etc.)		Medical therapies (orthodox) (extensive surgery, irradiation, cytotoxic drugs, etc.)
Immunotherapy (vaccines, gamma-globulins, thymus extract, etc.)		
Emotional support therapies (relaxation, visualisation, hypnosis, etc.)		Strong stress factors
Active life style (mental and physical)		Inactive life style
Fighting spirit		Stoic or accepting spirit

CHAPTER FOUR

ORTHODOXY: WHY THE EXPERTS FAIL

Modern orthodox medicine's treatment of cancer has involved the prolonged and devoted work of thousands of doctors and their helpers. Concerned physicians and surgeons, deeply troubled by the horrors of the disease that they see attack countless patients, have done everything in their power to stem its progress and restore health. The demoralising failure in case after case has not stopped them trying, ever harder, ever more strenuously. In some small areas there have been some notable successes.

Unfortunately it has to be admitted that in most areas, especially those of the major killing cancers, success has been at best marginal, usually absent and sometimes even a negative feature. The anticancer methods now being employed for the most part simply don't work. After half a century in some instances like skilled surgery, and a quarter of a century in the case of irradiation and chemotherapy, what these three orthodox methods have shown is that they fail almost every doctor and patient, however they are applied.

There is nothing surprising about that. As we shall see, they are not very good methods anyway. What is more, the history of human progress has always been dotted with good ideas which for one reason or another failed and were abandoned. What is remarkable about current treatments is that they have failed, but have not been abandoned. Indeed, they continue to be used with ever greater determination and enthusiasm.

This has to be a prime example of a triumph of faith over experience. It is almost as though some fire of hope is being kept alive that sooner or later these methods will achieve the success that has always been denied them. A parallel might be drawn with the military mentality of the Great War. It seemed so right to the established military

TC - D

37

opinion that ever more powerful mass attacks from allied to enemy
trenches were the correct way to breach the opposing defences, that
mass slaughter went on and on. Remorseless shelling and decimating
casualties failed to shake the opinion.

Now we have the sad state of affairs where the prongs of orthodox
attack, having totally failed to make any great impact on the incidence
or cure rate of cancer, are nevertheless still being applied more and more
vigorously.

If you pause to think, or if you discuss the matter with others, ask
yourself or them what the concept of cancer means. The usual response
to it is that it is a common disease which inevitably involves unpleasant
and unsuccessful therapies, followed by a decline to an often painful
death. That is average opinion in spite of the expenditure of monumental
amounts of money, time and research brain-power for several decades.

Do doctors think any differently? Do they see the diagnosis of
cancer as one which holds more than a remote glimmer of hope? Ask
them and see. Those who I have asked do not.

Then ask what the doctor would feel if he or one of his loved ones
developed a malignant cancer. Would he want to have extensive surgery,
painful and weakening radiation and cancer drugs, then a lingering death?
Or would he prefer to go quickly without being a burden to himself or
others? He will invariably choose the latter, albeit the choice is only
hypothetical. Most of his patients would make the same choice too.

Yet when he, or one of his cases does develop cancer, the whole
charade eventually gets re-played through to its near certain conclusion.
Here we encounter the anomalous situation of both doctor and patient
carrying out measures which they would not and do not objectively
choose. The logic would be curious if it were not so tragic.

Imagine for a moment a procedure in which the luckless victim
were anaesthetized while ill and in a condition of consequent weakness,
and during the anaesthetic his or her body was cut open and had parts of
it removed. As short a time after the operation as possible, the person is
exposed to several doses of nuclear emissions so that symptoms of
radiation sickness are suffered. Finally, sub-lethal amounts of drugs are
injected with horrifying side effects.

If this kind of villainy were perpetrated as a punishment on a child-
strangler or a mass-murderer, its degree of barbarity would still raise a
clamour of protest from every thinking person in the entire civilised
world. Carried out as an unsuccessful therapeutic measure in cases of
advanced cancer, on the other hand, seems to make it all right. Once
again the logic is of strange quality.

Today's orthodox cancer therapy in many ways is now coming very
close to malpraxis. Medical malpraxis is defined in the Gould Medical
Dictionary as "improper *or* injurious medical or surgical treatment

through carelessness, *ignorance* or intent" (my italics). Unquestionably contemporary treatment is injurious. There may be no ignorance displayed as the doctor is fairly confident of the result. But ignorance could also include ignorance of alternative, perhaps better ways.

Another authority[1] explains malpraxis more fully as being "The failure of employment of *reasonable* skill or *attention* on the part of a medical attendant thereby endangering the *health* or even the *life* of the patient" (my italics). Should not, I wonder, 'reasonable' attention include adequate heterodox knowledge? More certainly, should not the 'attention' include a guarantee of measures that should *reasonably* be expected to help, not, as in most cancer cases, a certainty of 'endangering' both the 'health' and the 'life' of the patient?

The same authority goes further to mention that "A more serious *criminal* lack of care arising from deliberate disregard for the care and *safety* of other persons (patients) constitutes *manslaughter*". Once again it does not seem unfair to pose the question, if a physician conducts a treatment that he knows jeopardises the safety of his patient, is that not deliberate? Could it not be criminal and thus manslaughter if the patient so treated dies of his treatment rather than of his disease? This is not a rhetorical question. Injury from treatment is invariable; threat to health and life is commonplace; death is frequent.

It is no longer a rarity to find patients at autopsy who have died, not of their cancers, but of the means used for treating them. This is not a theory. It is already a matter of widespread medical record. Opinion could quite reasonably see this state of affairs as legalised manslaughter. It is unthinkable that such an untenable situation could have been reached. Yet it exists.

These words should not in any way be regarded as a sweeping attack on all doctors. They are not the words of a disenchanted doctor whining at his colleagues. For doctors were trained from at least adolescence to accept established teaching more or less as dogma. They learn from their tutors and from their experience that nearly all their cancer cases die. They are taught to battle on with the recognised tools.

All this they do bravely and very often at much cost to their own health and morale. But what doctors are not taught to do, and for the most part do not therefore do, is question outside their trained-in parameters. Intelligent, doctors usually are. Subtle, skilled, persistent and deserving of love and trust they certainly can be. But innovative and imaginative, they usually are not.

It is essential at this point to jettison the entrenched view of the nature of cancer. Overboard too must go the idea that current therapeutic failure must either go on failing or go on at all. A tumour is

[1] Butterworth's *Medical Dictionary*.

not a disease. It is a prominent symptom of disease. When a cancer occurs it is not the tumour that is at fault, it is the entire body that is ill and thus letting the tumour grow. There is thus no point in attacking the tumour and weakening the body by undermining its defence methods at the same time. It is the body that must be restored to health. Everything about it must be aided, not harmed. Then resistance, retaliation and resurgence to sound health can start from inside.

That is how we must see the cancer problem from now on. And it is with that in mind that we must now direct cancer therapy in a totally different direction.

An example of the way in which orthodox therapy for cancer now exists more on hope than on conviction has been the recent excitement about interferon. Let it be said at once that if by some remote chance this preparation does turn out to be a cancer cure, it will be one of the greatest blessings ever. But what, in practical terms, are its chances?

Interferon is a defensive material produced in living tissues when they are attacked or 'stressed' by outside influences, notably viruses. Very quickly after attack, interferon-type compounds are produced. Their effect appears (so far) to be threefold: by acting as a bio-chemical burglar alarm to alert and encourage response in other cells, by producing antibodies that retard the growth of tumour cells, and by treating tumour cells as if they were invading viruses, thereby destroying or lysing them. Interferon can be isolated from blood serum after viral attack. As this natural material has already been shown to have some anti-tumour effect in experimental work, colossal expenditure is now being made on factories to manufacture a synthetic copy.

Hopes may now be fading, as some experts have already expressed serious doubts. In spite of popular acclaim and a press coverage almost unequalled in medical history, early results are disappointing. It has already been explained in the *British Medical Journal*[2] that results so far obtained are no better than by conventional radiation or chemotherapy (. . . and *they* are certainly not very good). One kind of cancer tested, myeloma, did worse than with standard chemotherapy. A group of lung cancer cases treated in New York showed precisely no response at all. Another group of breast cancer cases treated, who appeared at first to be showing some response, were later found more likely to be responding to pre-interferon treatment by other means.

The report's author concluded that although interferon preparations are still exciting to cancer specialists, the media have exaggerated the therapeutic importance. Others have warned about being misled. The tragic case of a little boy, Nicky Ellis, was reported in the national

---

[2] Sikora, Dr. K., Medical Research Council's Clinical Oncology Unit, Cambridge, UK, *B.M.J.*, No. 6244, Vol. 281, 1980.

press[3]. His parents, with extreme devotion, sold up their home and put the £27,000 proceeds with the father's redundancy pay and money collected by workmates to buy 'the wonder drug'. At that time Mr. Gordon Piller, Director of the Leukaemia Research Fund, appealed to parents not to take this kind of action as "Interferon on its own is not a treatment". (Nicky Ellis, weakened by several years of orthodox therapy to the extent that only at the age of 11 years was he changing from milk teeth to permanent teeth, failed to receive interferon. He succumbed during 1980.)

A summary of several opinions published in 1980[4] stressed that hopes should not be prematurely raised by irresponsible reporting. Interferon, it is concluded, is an interesting substance that may have value, but which is at present of major importance only as a subject of research. Others have gone further[5]. After a trial on a small number of cases, all patients showed side effects like appetite loss, anaemia, reduced white blood cell count, raised blood pressure and emotional confusion. The bottom line comes from the American Society of Clinical Oncology, which has publicly stated that there is "no evidence *or even remote* suggestion" (my italics) that interferon cures advanced cancer.

Setting aside the interferon saga there are really only four components of current orthodox cancer therapy. The first of these, hyperbaric oxygen (the use of oxygen at higher than normal pressure) has received little publicity. It depends on the belief, which is supported by considerable evidence, that a high concentration must be bad for tumour cells, as a low level is known to encourage them.

Oxygen normally dissolves in blood up to a maximum of only 0.3 ml of oxygen per 100 ml of blood at a pressure of 100 mm of mercury. By increasing the pressure to three atmospheres this can be increased twenty-fold to 6 ml per 100 ml. The pressure rise can be maintained in a special room or cannister. This kind of therapy is known to be of value in cases of oxygen shortage, some kinds of respiratory distress, or cyanide or smoke poisoning. Prime medical opinion[6] states that in spite of the popularity of this treatment in such cases it has "no *proved* merit in treatment of ageing, or impotence" (my italics). What it does not say is that it has no merit in the treatment of cancer. Indeed, there is an aim in the Gentle Method to increase tissue oxygenation in a number of ways. What is more, many people find episodes of exposure to hyperbaric oxygen to be re-invigorating if not rejuvenating. If cancer cells thrive best on a low oxygen level it would seem unwise to

[3] *Daily Express*, Monday 24.8.80, p. 7.

[4] Ridgeway, R., *Brit. Med. Assoc. Review*, Sept. 1980, p. 18 *et seq.*

[5] *Pulse*, 6 Sept. 1980, p. 27.

[6] Cecil, *Textbook of Medicine*, 1979.

lose any of the possible value of high pressure oxygen in cancer therapy, especially as this is a painless and non-dangerous form of treatment.

The qualities of being painless and non-dangerous cannot be ascribed to the three other main methods of orthodox cancer management. Indeed, the reverse. For all three are extremely painful and invariably extremely dangerous. Small wonder that the horrific triumvirate of surgery, radiation and chemotherapy have acquired the pejorative appellation of the 'cut-burn-poison' method.

In spite of the horrors that accompany their application, there is a certain amount of logic in their use according to contemporary established opinion. If cancer is a lump in the body that can get bigger or spread, some obvious combatting principles present themselves. As much as possible of the tumour should be cut out or off. As there may already have been some spread, try to get at what could not be removed, by exposing undiscovered cells to radiation. Finally, as there may still be isolated pockets of malignant cells, inject drugs into the blood stream so that they can be carried to those cells by the blood and, there, attack and kill them.

It is hard to oppose those as good sense measures. But they are based on the premise that the tumour is the disease. As the premise is wrong, apparently logical deductions from it are also likely to be wrong. There is no blame to be attached because of attempts to succeed along these lines. They seem obvious and logical. They are also the ingrained teaching principle of modern doctors. But the path that once appeared so promising has long since turned out to be a dead end.

What is remarkable is that so few have spotted the fact. They have missed the point that effort to make progress is now greater than ever, but progress itself is minute.

Surgery is of a standard that has never been equalled before. It is possible to reattach severed limbs, by-pass blocked arteries with grafts, transplant hearts and kidneys, as everyday procedures. Bigger, better and more accurately focussed radiation sources are available even in quite small district hospitals. Anti-neoplastic drugs in larger doses and infinite varieties of combination are in use.

It does appear unreasonable, with all these advantages and the near limitless funds, that progress must be going on by leaps and bounds. Yet it isn't. Because medicine has, quite simply, lost its way. The warnings are not all new.

*   *   *   *   *

Surgery is the oldest orthodox method now in use. From the earliest records there are descriptions of the amputation of limbs afflicted with what sound like tumours. Until quite recently, internal surgery was seldom attempted in view of the pain and the failure rate. The arrival of anaesthetics and aseptic methods to prevent or control infection, encouraged huge strides forward of surgical technique and skill.

Unquestionably surgery must, at this stage, still be regarded as an important aspect of cancer therapy. However, surgeons being as they are, things sometimes get out of hand, as when massive surgical procedures are undertaken in the mistaken belief that the more extensive the surgery, the better the result. The operation of radical mastectomy is an example of this. Until quite recent times, a breast malignancy was treated not only by removal of the breast, but also the muscles beneath it right down to the rib cage. The wound was continued up into the armpit which was dissected out and had parts of it, particularly the glands, removed. The surgical shock to the patient was enormous. The disfigurement was hideous. The success rate was very small. Even before the Second World War some eminent surgeons had abandoned this operation[7]. There are now doubts even about the value of a far smaller scale operation For, as Tobias recently summarised[8], "... it is *not known* whether local surgical removal is necessary, though this is *usually recommended*" (my italics). After a century of trying it is still "not known" ... but it is being done just the same!

Removal of a tumour by surgical means does have one distinct advantage, even according to heterodox principles. Massive and active tumours appear able to exert an overwhelming influence which inhibits the body's natural defences[9].

This being said, surgery must only be permitted in a limited number of instances. There is no question of removing the tumour simply because it is there. Size may be a reason by virtue of defence-inhibition. Or a tumour could be having a mechanical effect that is jeopardizing life itself perhaps by pressing on vital organs and causing obstruction, and so on. However, except in these latter instances, surgery should never be regarded as an emergency or even urgent matter.

There are some conditions recognised as pre-cancerous. Some polyps, bulging tags of skin found in the nose, uterus or rectum, are of that nature. So are papillomata, small fronds of tissue that grow inside the bladder. So too are heavily pigmented moles on the skin. A very serious pre-cancerous state is that of hyperplasia or speeding-up of growth on the neck of the womb, often located by taking cervical smears.

Surgical removal of such lesions as these is a wise precaution. What

[7] Keynes, G., *Brit. Med. Journal*, 2, p. 632, 1937.

[8] Tobias, J.S., Mastectomy, *World Medicine*, 6 Oct. 1979, p. 47.

[9] Norman, S.J., Schardt, M. and Sorkin, E., *Proc. Eures. Symp. on Macrophages and Cancer*.

is more, the extent of the surgery required is such that there is seldom any great shock to the patient, and recovery is swift and untroubled.

Tumours of the womb are also, as a rule, very slow growing, Thus, if detected early in its life, removal of the womb (hysterectomy) as a non-urgent procedure may well prevent trouble later as no spread beyond the womb is likely.

More damage can be done to patients by premature surgery than there are benefits so obtained. Surgical procedures on ill people are strongly counter-productive. It is better to wait a while, building the patient up to the best possible condition by techniques comprising the Gentle Method. Then, and only then, is essential surgery carried out. The preparation period more than compensates for the delay.

I stress that to operate in undue haste, on a case of malignancy, and before adequate promotion of the patient's general health has been achieved, is positively contra-indicated.

What is more, no surgery should ever be regarded as a cure of cancer. At the very best it may have removed a tumour. The underlying causes of that tumour may well still operate. False sense of security should never be encouraged. And full supportive anti-cancer regimes should always be adopted. Otherwise cancer is very likely to recur.

If there are some points to be made in favour of surgery, there are very few good things to be said about the second principle orthodox weapon, radiation. It is nearly always bad, even if there appear to be some temporary benefits. There are a small number of tumours, nominally those of the skin and some embryonic tissues, which are highly susceptible, or radio-sensitive. These are the only cases on which radiation should be used, ever. In nearly every other instance more harm than good is done.

Radiation is used because it is fatal to living cells. Cells which receive above a certain amount will succumb. This is why great care is taken to protect those who work with radiation. This is why many of those exposed to nuclear blasts died. The condition caused is known as radiation sickness. Some kinds of cells, notably the more primitive, embryonic tissue-resembling cells, are more sensitive to radiation than are the more mature cells. Similarly, malignant cells are more sensitive than healthy ones, in that they are destroyed by small radiation dosage.

The aim of radiation therapy is a kind of controlled radiation sickness. Narrow beams of radiation are passed through the body so as to affect the tumour. By careful focussing of the beam, and by moving it about, it can be directed through different parts of the body, but always at such an angle that the tumour is in the path of the rays. In this way it is sought to give the tumour a higher dose than healthy zones elsewhere.

Unfortunately, the technique leaves a lot to be desired for accuracy. To start with, the exact position of the tumour is only known to a degree. Also it has no precise boundaries. So, radiation in too high a dose can easily affect healthy neighbouring tissues, while not all tumour cells necessarily get a fatal dose. To expand the target area is to kill off or damage more and more healthy cells.

There are other problems. Radiation not only destroys cells altogether. It is one of the things that can bring about somatic mutation in healthy cells, as discussed in the previous chapter. Consequently radiation given at the wrong stage can worsen a patient's chances[10].

Amongst cells which are highly radio-sensitive are those of the immune system, the glands and the bone marrow. Yet it has already been explained that these are the very cells on which the main part of natural defences against cancer depends. So, by irradiating a tumour, there is often produced a most dangerous suppression of, and injury to, the tissues most needed for survival.

A few years ago, during a discussion on unorthodox therapies, there came an interesting pronouncement[11]. A senior, establishment cancer authority stated that in the evaluation of anti-tumour affect only objective decrease in the size of the measurable lesions can be accepted as evidence. There is an obvious error here. In some tumours the malignant cells are not always the most radio-sensitive. If such a tumour is irradiated, more healthy cells than malignant ones will die. As cells die the tumour shrinks in size, thereby satisfying the criterion of the pronouncement above. But what is left of the tumour can well be more dangerous than before as the proportion of malignant cells it contains will now be higher[12].

One more fact needs to be mentioned about radiation. At the same time as it depletes bodily resistance it brings about the distressing symptoms of radiation sickness. General feelings of being ill, bad appetite, nausea, lassitude and weakness are just some of these. Coming alone they are bad enough. Coming quickly after the trauma of major surgery they are little short of torture.

One of the most incisive attacks on the use of radiation came unwittingly from a report on the treatment of children with brain tumours[13]. A group of cases were found to have suffered from brain exposure to radioactivity to the extent that they had diminished intelligence, decrease in memory ability, impaired mathematical skills, permanent personality changes, heightened anger, depression and

[10] Livingston, Dr. R., University of Texas, testifying before *Frontiers of Cancer Research* hearing, US House Select Committee on Aging.

[11] Hurley, D.J., and others, Human lymphocyte-tumour cell interaction, *JAMA*, Vol. 241, No. 24, p. 2631 *et seq.*, 1979.

[12] Report to the Legislature by the California Cancer Advisory Council, p. 57.

[13] Zwartjes, Dr. W.J., Children's Hospital, Denver, USA, reported in *Medical News*, 3 April 1980, p. 8.

introversion. No less than three-quarters of those treated with radiation underwent such impairment compared with only one-fifth of cases that had avoided irradiation. Several had been committed to mental institutions. Quite rightly, the reporting doctor said, "the psychological costs for these individuals are thus very high, and call into question whether survival under such circumstances is really worth the tremendous cost". (The kinds of cost he had in mind were not specified.)

Perhaps the case is, in a way, gratifying. It showed that in the minds of Senior Physicians, at last, the results of such treatment of child cancer patients are now raising doubts about the quality of life of the survivors. I should think so too!!!

But of all the great weapons of contemporary cancer treatment, infinitely the most dreadful is the use of chemotherapeutic drugs. In many respects the reasons for their use is because of their high toxicity. They are amongst the most toxic drugs known. These drugs can undoubtedly kill cells. Malignant cells are very susceptible to their effects. The principle then is much like that of radiation, to kill the tumour cells and leave the healthy ones. It sounds simple. But it isn't. For the dose is critical, the difference between enough to kill malignant cells and that fatal to healthy ones is exceedingly narrow. What is more, again like radiation, these drugs are as well-known for their ability to cause malignancy as they are for their curative capacity. Additionally, they further suppress the body's immune system, thus further limiting a healthy response to the disease.

Of all things, though, it is the side effects of chemotherapy that are most dreadful to the patient. These include nausea, vomiting, bone marrow damage, bleeding, increased infections, loss of hair, liver and kidney damage, numbness, impotence, sterility, scarring of lungs, shortness of breath, weakness, fall in blood pressure, diarrhoea, sores in mouth, skin rashes, fever, sensitivity to sunlight, loss of consciousness, violent allergic reactions, phlebitis, disorientation, lethargy, bladder irritation, heart damage, skin ulcerations, pigmentation of nail beds, loss of balance, visual disturbance, difficulty in walking, pigmentation of the skin, mental confusion, muscle spasms and death.

Death is an unwelcome 'side effect', but it is the others that prove the most insufferable.

It is not as though the cytotoxic drugs even bring about cure. In the case of tumours of the alimentary tract, which account for 27% of all recorded malignancies in the United Kingdom[14], the overall survival rate for five years is less than one in ten. These depressing figures have not altered for a number of years despite the introduction of cytotoxic

[14] James, R.D., *J. Royal Soc. Medicine*, Vol. 73, Sept. 1980, p. 659.

agents.

Furthermore, an assessment of combined chemotherapy in the treatment of breast cancer[15] indicates that this has not produced any improvement in overall survival of patients, and may, in fact, shorten the time of survival of certain patients who already have spread of the disease. The combined chemotherapy in non-responders to treatment "... not only seems to shorten their survival, but adversely affects the quality of what life they do have, due to the side effects of these very toxic agents".

Here is raised, for me, one of the main tenets expressed in this book. Far more important than extending the length of the lifespan, is improving the quality of that span. It is this that has been forgotten in the annals of cancer treatment. To the vast majority of people it is much more important to live out their remaining time in comfort and happiness than to eke out an extra spell like an aged, sick and tired dog.

If this principle is kept in mind it becomes difficult to explain why cancer therapy relies upon widespread surgery, the deliberate use of radiation that damages resistance, and an ultimate attack with drugs on the defensive immune system. This simply cannot all be being done with the object of restoring health, for everyone knows it does not.

The trouble is that the main aim of medicine is being overlooked. This is why I claim, in this aspect of cancer therapy, that medicine has lost its way. The aim always was, and should be, not mere life, but life free from pain and having the quality of being enjoyable.

Orthodoxy has taken a wrong turning and led medicine, its practitioners and their patients, by the nose along it. And orthodoxy has a fearful grip. This is witnessed by the phenomenon we see every day when, in spite of the known, dismal failure rates and hazards of treatment, people persevere with the methods. These are not just the poor or the stupid that so persevere. Wealthy and influential people, heads of Government, film stars, and senior members of the medical professions too, still go on dying of malignancy and the effects of its treatment. That such people continue to die is surely commentary enough on the efficacy of the methods?

*   *   *   *   *

After such drastic and incessant failure, it becomes hard to comprehend why not just patients, but all doctors too, are not wide-eyed and open-eared in the hunt for alternative, more successful methods. It is not as if these are unavailable, as we shall see.

One problem is that the existing system, albeit a bad one, is a

[15] *Lancet*, 1980, Vol. 1, No. 8168, p. 580.

familiar and thus, in its way, a comforting and comfortable one. There are more patients who do not want to live, than most folk would expect. For such people succumbing to cancer is a socially acceptable and morally guilt-free means of suicide.

The doctor too finds his role a secure one. No-one expects more of him than that he goes through the standard rigmarole. This accomplished, no blame for the misery or the death attaches to him. If he tried an unorthodox method and, even after a period of success, it failed, he could find himself the object of litigation. As long as he sticks to orthodox methods of certain failure, he is totally safe.

Although one does not necessarily approve of these explanations they are at least understandable. What is less understandable is the dogged resistance of the majority of doctors to the existence of alternative methods. And not only are these denied. Even the parts of alternative techniques such as the Gentle Method, which are of obvious common sense and which, when tried, have such obviously beneficial results, are resisted. To a large extent they are even totally excluded from therapy. One treatment, the use of amygdalin (or, under its trade name Laetrile), has been the subject of vehement language, litigation and prison sentences in the USA. On both sides there have been arguments with bad reasoning, emotional outbursts, unprofessional wrangling, indiscretions and discrepancies. A vituperative atmosphere which helps no-one has resulted.

Now, there are points for and against the use of amygdalin. In my opinion the pros overwhelmingly outweigh the cons. Nevertheless one can understand some physicians harbouring doubts and reluctance. (Though these are usually swiftly overcome by trying it on a case or two.) It so happens that amygdalin is an important component of the Gentle Method. Reluctant physicians can, if they choose, omit it. But there are no such doubts to be harboured over other parts of the Method. High vitamin intake, mineral adjustments and supplements, emotional support and, above all, dietary factors, can have no counter arguments. They are plain common sense.

However ill a person is, they *do* help. There is no question about it. They *even* help patients who are being done to death by the cut, burn and poison technique. Yet, some doctors cannot, or will not, see or try them even as such support methods.

This is pig-headed, ignorant cruelty and is contrary not only to Hippocratic teaching but to the Hippocratic Oath itself.

There is little to be gained by going into the 'Laetrile controversy' to any depth. What emerges from it is that here is a long-known substance with an alleged beneficial effect. This latter is contested, as is the claim that it is of very low toxicity.

Clearly, if amygdalin (sometimes even more confusingly called

Vitamin B-17) is beneficial and of low toxicity, then it can prove highly advantageous. So what of these two factors? To start with, more or less nothing is truly non-toxic. Amygdalin, when taken by mouth, is hydrolysed in the stomach and some of it is converted to a cyanide compound. Not all such compounds are bad. In small amouts cyanide is required as a component of the essential erythropoietic vitamin B-12. Large doses of hydrolysed amygdalin could prove injurious.

This was shown in a series of tests in USA, in which experimental dogs were fed the substance. So far, so good. When the dogs died, this was claimed as a demonstration of how dangerous amygdalin is to humans. What was not pointed out was that excessive doses were administered, and of already fermented amygdalin which was thus high in cyanide. The same could be said of many other substances. Three or four pounds of sugar might be tolerated by a human over a few hours. Fermented to alcohol, the same amount could prove fatal. Also, even doses of safe drugs, if widely exceeded, could cause death. The right, small amount of digoxin will slow the racing heart. Ten times the correct dose may well stop it altogether.

Anyway, to be at its most effective amygdalin should be given by intravenous injection. By this route the problems of hydrolysis are unlikely to occur. I personally have given hundreds of injections of ten grams at a time and have never seen a side effect more severe than a mild and brief rigor.

It is of interest that there exists in the USA an official Registry of Toxic Effects of Chemical Substances. In the 1976 edition, published by the US Department of Health, Education and Welfare, there is no mention of either amygdalin or laetrile; this, although the purported objective of the volume is " . . . to identify all known toxic substances which may exist in our environment . . .".

One widely used classification of toxicity[16] grades substances from Class 6 (supertoxic), through Class 2 (slightly toxic), to Class 1 (practically non-toxic). According to this, amygdalin falls between 1 and 2. Saccharin falls between Classes 3 and 4 (moderate to very toxic). Cytotoxic drugs belong in Classes 5 and 6. So much for amygdalin toxicity. The summary is that, administered correctly, it is very, very safe. An observation borne out by my own experience.

Even more unfair has been the wrangle over the efficacy of amygdalin. Wild claims for its success have been made which have led to extortion, chicanery and charlatanism. Unprofessional counterclaims have been even worse. One example was the work of one of the most senior scientists of the last fifty years, Professor Kanematsu Sigiura,who died at a great age in 1980. The Sloan-Kettering Institute's publicised

[16] Casarett and Doull, *Toxicology*, MacMillan Publishing, New York, 1975.

report on one of Sigiura's experiments stated, " . . . there clearly was *no benefit* in the leukaemia". Yet Sigiura's own report on the same experiment (on amygdalin), and which was deliberately leaked, said the opposite. "This indicates that amygdalin had a *certain* inhibitory action on the development of leukaemia . . . ". (My italics in both quotations.)

Who is one to believe? The impeccable integrity of Sigiura or the highly-esteemed Institute? I cannot answer that question, though in my research for this volume I came across the interesting detail that as an example of possible bias one could not forbear to mention that one James Fisk, who is or was a director of the huge pharmaceutical concern Lederle Laboratories, was at one point Chairman of the Board of the Sloan-Kettering Institute.

Prejudiced reporting (both ways) clouds the issues. Writing a legal comment for a leading American medical publication[17], an author applauded a court decision against Laetrile because it "stops the nonsense". In the article he mentioned the sad case of a boy, Chad Green, who " . . . died of leukaemia in Mexico after being taken there . . . for Laetrile therapy . . .". It is easy to misread from this that Chad died *because* of the Laetrile. There is no such evidence. From all accounts, the boy was already desperately ill at least partly because of the orthodox therapy he had already had.

In 1977 a leading proponent of amygdalin and other alternative cancer treatment methods forecast three things. Two of those have already come about. He said that amygdalin would be legalised in the USA. So far the State of Kentucky was the 22nd to put such legality on the Statute. The second prophecy was that there would be a full scale clinical trial of amygdalin under properly controlled conditions. A new trial has recently been announced[18]. Some doubts must still be harboured as it is to be conducted by the US National Cancer Institute.

Personally I wish such a trial could be financed in the United Kingdom. Far away from the battlefields, it might be more free from either side's bias.

In most European countries amygdalin has never been illegal. This is not surprising as it is extracted mostly from bitter almond. Bitter almond, cherry and peach, all sources of amygdalin preparations, have been in use for the treatment of tumours by European physicians for at least two millenia[19]. Famous names that have used them abound. Celsus in ancient Rome used almond to treat 'putrid flesh'. Largus, another Roman, used it for bladder tumours. Galen, who influenced medicine for

[17]Curran, W.J., Law-medicine notes, *New Eng. J. Med.*, Vol. 302, No. 11, 13 March 1980, p. 619.
[18]*Doctor*, 20 Nov. 1980, p. 32.
[19]Hartwell, J.L., Survey of plants for US Nat. Cancer Institute.

over forty generations, used almonds for 'scirrhus of the liver'. Pliny the Elder mentions almond oil in the treatment of condylomata. Avicenna also used the oil for tumours of uterus, spleen, stomach and liver. There are plenty of other records up into the late nineteenth century, of doctors using the amygdalin-containing substances as anti-tumour agents. At a time when so many old ideas are being resurrected and retried, it might be as well for those who are as yet ignorant of the use of amygdalin to await reliable assessment. Those who do not have first hand experience should keep their mouths closed until they know what they are talking about.

*　　　*　　　*　　　*　　　*

Quite surely there is a vast amount of work still to be done regarding cancer. Existing methods should continue to be investigated either to look for success, or to prove their worthlessness and put an end to their use. There should, however, be a readjustment of research time and funds with less being spent on largely unsuccessful methods, and more on the search for newer ideas.

For example, the psychosomatic element needs far more study. Numerous workers for over a century have pointed the way and proclaimed the importance of such factors in cancer causation and treatment. Gendron[20] in 1701, Burrows[21] in 1783, Nunn in 1822, Walshe[22] in 1846, the famous Sir James Paget[23], describer of Paget's disease, in 1879, Snow[24] in 1893, and Elida Evans[25] in 1922, are the names of just a few prominent signposts. It is time for some at least to look along the routes indicated. Every doctor can recall patients who have, with the help of determination, lived far longer than expected. Others have awaited a special event only to deteriorate and die without a struggle a few days later.

A recent book on the subject[26] has shown that this entire concept is far from dead. A review for the Royal Society of Medicine[27] advises quite unequivocally that "It is a book that all doctors should read and reflect on . . .". I can think of no better advice.

There is no other way to summarise orthodoxy in cancer therapy

[20] Gendron, D., *Enquiries into the Nature, Knowledge and Cure of Cancers*, p. 72. London, 1701.

[21] Burrows, J., *A Practical Essay on Cancer*, p. 25. London, 1783.

[22] Walshe, W.H., *Nature and Treatment of Cancer*, p. 155. London, 1846.

[23] Paget, Sir James, *Surgical Pathology*, p. 800. London, 1870.

[24] Snow, Herbert, *Cancers and the Cancer-Process*, p. 34. London, 1893.

[25] Evans, Elida, *A Psychological Study of Cancer*, p. 126. New York, 1926.

[26] Stoll, B.A., *Mind and Cancer Progress*. John Wiley, Chichester, 1979.

[27] Twycross, R.G., *J. Royal Soc. Medicine*, Vol. 73, May 1980, p. 396.

than to state, without prejudice and merely with dispassionate observation, that it is totally unsatisfactory. When, with the benefit of vast resources, the cream of medical and scientific brain-power has been applied to the problem for half a century with scarcely any success, then unsatisfatory is a mild word to describe the situation.

Some promising signs are to be noted in all fairness. The chances of people surviving for five years with leukaemia is now three times as good as it was twenty years ago. Now it is almost 20%![28]

But some people are growing far more vociferous in their complaints and their choice of language. Professor Eric Wilkes was reported[29] for a paper he delivered on Cancer Management. One can do no better than to quote him at some length. He made his opinion clear that much of cancer management was "lousy medicine". Commenting further:—

> "Despite the multiplicity of treatments now available, the natural history of most cancers has been only slightly modified by these incredibly expensive and large-scale efforts. Of course marvellous breakthroughs have been achieved in chemotherapy with childhood leukaemias, Hodgkin's disease, chorionic carcinomas and testicular neoplasms. But there is an enormous amount of cytotoxic therapy being used on solid tumours, where the only outcome you can predict is that it will be no damn good.
>
> "Cytotoxic drugs are often doing more to prolong patients dying than to prolong their living. They are often used wastefully, with poor clinical judgment, and to give the doctor a role when he can think of nothing else to do for the patient."

Speaking of patients entering his terminal care hospice, he said:—

> " . . . a lot of patients want to come to St. Luke's because they have chemophobia. They know they are not going to be cured, but they are less afraid of dying than of being given yet another nasty infusion from which it will take them two weeks to recover before it is time for the next lot."

And as a summary,

> "When ablative surgery has failed, the patient is scared, the radiotherapists have shone their rays, the physician thinks: 'What can we do?'—and comes up with the answer 'Let's try something—mycin'. As a placebo, this is expensive, and disastrous medicine."

[28] *Cancer Statistics: Survival.* H.M. Stationery Office.
[29] *Pain Topics*, June 1980, p. 8.

Consternation is most obviously justified. Cancer mortality overall is increasing so that it is the only major cause of death which has continued to rise from 1900 through 1976.[30]

This in spite of the use of treatments that terrify the recipients and which go on and on failing. One American physician[31] has foretold the future as he sees it. He says, "there will be a medical edition of the Nuremberg Trials. The atrocities now being committed in the name of orthodox medicine, the suppression of life-giving scientific data, the needless loss of lives, mutilation of bodies, and excessive suffering, ... will not continue to be tolerated .... Ultimately, these criminals and their political lackeys will be brought to trial ...".

Those may sound harsh words to British ears. Here it will be thought of as enough if those in authority merely remove their blinkers and mend their ways. More moderate views will triumph if Mr. Ian Kennedy, Reader in Law at King's College, London, has his way. Speaking on BBC radio[32] he said "Medical schools must simply be dragged back into our world and out of their hermetically sealed cocoon in which we [the patients] are counters with which the game of life is played. The principles by reference to which doctors act must be the product of general discussion and debate. We must take over."

Such a reasoned revolution is inevitable if doctors go on with such demonstrable failures as contemporary cancer therapy. Doctors will lose the status that they largely deserve and which is vital to the successful practice of medicine, if they go on letting their people down by deliberate blindness and dogged reluctance. The loss will be to both doctors and to patients if the art is so blemished.

*　　　*　　　*　　　*　　　*

I challenge anyone to show sound evidence that, for example, a random group of advanced breast tumour patients do better when considered as a whole, or even live longer, on surgery, deep x-ray, and chemotherapy, than they do when left totally untreated. In my experience they don't.

So what should the individual do when faced with the decision as to what kind of treatment to accept, ... and everyone has the inalienable right to such a choice? Certainly nothing in this book should be construed as advice to them not to undergo orthodox methods. These methods are widely recommended by, and undergone by, doctors. A

---

[30] Schneiderman, Dr. M., Assoc. Director of US National Cancer Institute, to Senate Health Sub-Committee, 1979.

[31] Halstead, B.W., *Amygdalin Therapy*, p. 40, 1977.

[32] Reith Lectures, No. 4, 1980.

great breakthrough and the long sought-after success may be just around the corner.

Every sufferer should, if possible, find out the exact nature of his or her diagnosis. The next ideal step would be to visit a cancer ward, see such similar cases, and note the results of their treatment. Then the available statistics on success and failure should be carefully read.

On the one hand is the offer of painful treatment, an undignified decline and very low chances of success. On the other, unorthodox methods, in my opinion, offer painless treatment, vastly improved feelings of well being, and at least the same chance of success.

Both my family and I have long since made our own decisions.

CHAPTER FIVE

UNORTHODOXY: PEOPLE, OPINIONS AND CASES

All over the world people are working on the unorthodox yet realistic approaches to cancer control. More and more are being converted to such promising methods as their faith, hope and patience with the failing orthodox techniques recede.

Twenty years ago there were just a few intrepid voices like those of Gerson and Issels. Now there are dozens. Soon there will be hundreds and thousands.

It should prove interesting and, I hope, useful to discuss some workers, past and present, to learn of their ideas and methods, which, although seemingly different, all lead to similar conclusions and, most important of all, to greater rates of success than other methods.

There are of course far too many to receive proper space and credit. There are doctors like Alec Forbes, Ian Pearce, Dorothy West, Malcolm Carruthers, Ernesto Contreras, Bruce Halstead, John Richardson, Oscar Todd, Lockie, Simnett and Kilsby, and others too numerous to mention. Similarly, there are growing numbers of lay therapists like Norman Eddie, Pearl Coleman, Leon Chaitow, Maureen Gallington, and the Gerson-Straus family. While not allowed to treat cancer themselves and alone, they are able to give the valuable advice of their disciplines to those who are in charge of such cases.

Then there are the non-medical organisers and teachers like Sir George Trevelyan, Marcus and Marika McCauseland, Michael Wheatley and Frank Hourigan. There are helpful organisations like the McCarrison Society, the Pure Water Preservation Society, Health for the New Age, and many many more.

They will all, I am sure, forgive me for selecting just a few people to discuss in detail, while sharing the praise with each and every one.

*   *   *   *   *

If ever a man deserved the title of gentleman by virtue of being a gentle man, as well as by being man enough to stand up and speak out, often alone, for his principles, and if ever that double honour were found in the same person as a loved, honoured, and immensely capable physician, then the final product might well be named Dr. Hans Moolenburgh.

This is the man, then a family doctor in Haarlem, Holland, who saw the dangers of orthodox cancer therapy a couple of decades ago. Not only that, but having criticised it to the point of drawing opprobium and ostracism from his colleagues, he set about searching the avenues of "fringe medicine" for some hope of an alternative. After he had found the first few hopeful ideas and techniques, it was he who built them into a programme that could be used by non-medical people. He had little choice in this, for medical people would not use them anyway.

He it was who coined the name 'The Gentle Method' for the techniques he was using. Although the name now has come to encompass a much broader field, albeit of techniques, many of which are used by him, he it was who first conceived of the idea that cancer treatment did not need to be filled with pain, fear, weakening side effects and, almost always, failure. He felt, practised, and taught that there were other gentler ways, ways that suited his own kindly, warm, humane and gentle nature. The Gentle Method owed is nascence to this exceedingly gentle man.

Moolenburgh believes very strongly in the psychological and spiritual aspects of life in general and of cancer management in particular. He says, shrewdly, that he never saw a cancer patient who was healed and who was the same person afterwards. Further, he feels that unless the sufferer changes, there is a very big chance indeed that the tumour will take over the whole of the body's power.

Speaking of repressed facets of personality, denied expression because they were unacceptable to those who educated us, he reminds that these repressed characteristics do not die or go away. His concept is that they can find their preserved, vigorous, youthful expression in later life in the form of aggressive, ruthless cancer. Only if they can be reintegrated does the uncontrolled cancer form of expression diminish as being no longer necessary. Once again the change in the whole person is a manifest part of the cure of their malignancy.

He quotes[1] a case which demonstrates his views. (Readers are

---

[1] Personal communication to the author, 27 Sept. 1980.

reminded that Dutch-speaking Hans Moolenburgh writes this comment in English, in which he has a fluently expressive and individual style.)

"A female patient in her mid fifties is operated on for a cancer in the breast. Her general condition is not good, she suffers from severe depressions and feeling that she would like to 'let go' as so many of our cancer patients show, either openly or in the depth. She comes to me for non toxic cancer treatment, for that gentle, non aggressive method that is coveted by so many patients nowadays. Though she is doing exactly as I tell her, and obediently swallows all vitamins and minerals I give her, her general condition is not improving and she has that dead tiredness that broods ill for cancer patients. I now begin a series of talks with her and it appears that deep down, where she had not told it even to herself, she is exasperated by her very difficult friend who lives with her in the same house. Now this ladyfriend is indeed a very difficult person to live with, but my patient, a very Christian lady, has told herself that she must never make a row, always be understanding, always be gentle, never fight back.

"Her father has taught her this lifestyle and it is so ingrained in her personality that it is impossible for me to alter her submissive attitude. As a matter of fact my patient was slowly being killed by her friend, and I looked on helplessly. But then, as the weeks went on, and later on as the months and even years went on, there was a change in my patient. She slowly detected how, without actually making a row, she could look at the tantrums of her friend with a sort of friendly detachment, like you look at a difficult but beloved child. There was a diminishment and at last a vanishing of hate, and there was a realisation that what she had experienced from her friend was the same she had experienced from a rather difficult mother. Always, because of Christian love, real difficulties in her parental home had been smoothed over, forgotten, not expressed. The attitude of the child in her had been brought over in her adult life and had slowly poisoned her, until at last the other personality, the lively and not so sweet smiling one, broke through in the cancer.

"As soon as she began to show that real detachment and that diminshment of hatred the therapy got going. It was as if until now the vitamins had just got in through the mouth and left with the stools, but now there was growing strength. The dead tiredness left her and at last she understood that there is another side to Christianity than sweet suffering gentleness: the cleansing of the temper with a whip. The Gentle Method eventually made her less gentle, but more of a whole person."

Moolenburgh was the first prominent teacher to come and lecture in England in 1978, on the Gentle Method. It is disturbing that he came not at the invitation of our august professional bodies. He came at the request of a far seeing and enlightened naturopath, Dr. Leon Chaitow, who invited him to his home, gave it over for the whole day to those of us who crowded there to hear, and to the best of my knowledge, got little thanks from anyone.

Nevertheless it was at Chaitow's home that the Gentle Method of Hans Moolenburgh was first taught in England. A point that reflects much credit on both.

The teacher summarises his views on cancer in this way.

> " . . . I would like to point out that a spiritually and psychologically non-changed cancer patient is a patient in danger. That the Gentle Method aims at more than control of the cancer and freedom from symptoms. That it aims at new persons, who really have been made new through the darkness of a terrible illness."

For my part it is not possible to over emphasize the particular debt I owe to this colleague for his example, his clinical ability and the learning he passed on so willingly.

*   *   *   *   *

Dr. Josef Issels is one of the great pioneers of unorthodox cancer medicine. Even now some of the ideas and principles he was teaching twenty years ago sound avant garde to many who encounter them for the first time.

In one of his major papers[2] he summarised a fifteen year survival follow-up of 750 of his cases. His very opening words were both an indictment and a warning of the sterility of existing methods.

> "About 20% of all patients suffering from cancer . . . live for five years or more after surgery, irradiation and chemo-therapy. Despite improvements in technique and chemo-therapy a decisive increase in this duration cannot be expected in the present state of knowledge."

As much as two decades earlier he had developed his

[2] Issels, J., Immunotherapy in progressive metastatic cancer, *Clinical Trials Journal*, London, 1970, Vol. 7, No. 3, pp. 357-366.

Ganzheitstherapie, whole body therapy, propounding the concept that successful treatment of many diseases, especially cancer, depended not on mere tumour-orientated methods but on restoring normal, healthy function to the body as a single complete unit.

His contemporary, Druckrey[3], had also stressed that cancer development became possible only by virtue of the diminishing of that 'natural resistance' which destroys the cancer cells normally and constantly arising in a seemingly healthy organism.

Issels regards cancer in basically the same way, after thirty further years of close scrutiny. The sequence of events of cancer development are listed as:

1. Causative factors (prenatal or hereditary, dietary, environmental, psychic, and the devitalising effects of infected toxic areas in the body). Any number of these lead to
2. Secondary damage, leading to
3. A 'tumour-forming' internal environment and lowered resistance, leading to
4. Tumour formation and continued growth, leading to
5. Tumour related symptoms.

The tumour itself is thus seen as a late stage of the disease able to arise and grow only in a bed already prepared for it.

And so many factors need to be combatted in any comprehensive approach to such a complex aetiological background, Issels devised his Combination Therapy, a programme having many similarities to the Gentle Method.

An early aspect of the Issels programme is to examine the body thoroughly for known, or more often, unsuspected foci of infection. Common offenders are sinus conditions, faulty teeth and gums, and chronically infected tonsils. Any such areas detected are corrected, if necessary, surgically. Emotional and psychic stresses are treated with appropriate mental support techniques. Diet is adjusted and vitamin and mineral preparations given.

Periods of fever, up to 105°F, are initiated by injection of bacterial preparations to stimulate the temperature control centre in the brain. Another method of achieving this is by microwave exposure, or sauna-type heat environments for up to ninety minute periods.

Haematogenic Oxidation Therapy (HOT) relies on removing up to 200 ml of the patient's blood, and after bubbling oxygen through it and irradiating it with ultraviolet rays, returning it to the circulation.

In common with the Gerson Method, a high potassium intake is

---

[3] Druckrey, H., *Med. Welt*, 1950, 1, 1613, 1652.

encouraged. Enzyme therapy is also a prominent feature of the method. Another similarity, this time with the studies of Dr. Jean Thomas, appears in the use of Immunological Therapy. After malignant growths have been liquefied and subjected to ultra-filtration in the laboratory, the resulting filtrate is cultured on a beef-agar medium. Having been re-inoculated into numerous fresh cultures for a long period to attenuate activity, and after rigorous animal tests for safety, the final product is re-injected. Closer perhaps to Thomas' work is the use of tissue specific anti-sera prepared from tumour extracts from other patients, and others similar to those used by Gerlach[4] in which the anti-sera are collected from horses immunised with cultures from human tumour products. Issels has pointed out that his method is useful in detecting previously undiscovered secondary growths as they reveal their involvement by pain and tenderness after immunotherapy.

It is understandable for a lone researcher to detect good work in his own results. However, Issels' cases were independently assessed[5] with remarkable results. It is stressed that all the cases assessed already had "progressive tumour growth with metastases and relapses after termination of 'normal', i.e. conventional, treatment". Patients who were alive and well after five years and who had had both conventional and immunotherapy rated 18%. Of those who had had only immuno-therapy 42 (26%) were alive and well. When compared with other reported series of cases (unrelated to Issels) these figures were dramatic, as in the other series the five year survival rates were only 9.5% (Schwaiger, 1955) and 5% (Rossolec, 1955), respectively. Furthermore, when the 42 immunotherapy cases were reassessed a further fifteen years later (1970), only two had died from late relapses of their cancer and one from an unconnected infectious meningitis. The other 39 showed no sign of cancer and remained "fully fit for work without any further follow-up treatment" during the intervening years.

In spite of this Issels has been thoroughly pilloried, including by legal action, by opponents of his methods. Nevertheless he remains at work in the famous Ringberg-Klinic in the town of Bad Wiesee in Bavaria. To some of us there are aspects of his theories which are, even now, innovative, bold and brilliant. Other aspects, like encouraging tumour elimination by irradiation and chemotherapy as well as by surgery[6] seem a conflict of two diametrically opposed and perhaps mutually exclusive principles. This is particularly unexpected in view of

---

[4] Gerlach, F. (1961) Immunobiologische Studien bei malignen Tumoren und Haemoblastosen, *Krebsarzt*, 2, xix, 54, and (1970) *Wiener Tierarztl.*

[5] Audier, A.G., *Die Medizinische*, No. 40, 1960.

[6] Issels, J., Immunotherapy in progressive metastatic cancer, *Clinical Trials Journal*, London, 1970, Vol. 7, No. 3, p. 360.

the figures quoted above which clearly show combination therapy to be better on its own.

Nevertheless, Issels has, for many years, treated cancer cases with a far greater measure of success than most can claim. One of the cases recorded in this chapter in some detail is his. And Mrs. Brohn speaks for herself as well as for Dr. Issels' success with her.

*   *   *   *   *

Dr. Hans Nieper, MD, has worked in many parts of the world, notably the United Kingdom, USA and, as now, in the Department of Medicine of the Silbersee Hospital in Langenhagen, West Germany.

The field of alternative medicine where it is applied to cancer has many people of heart, fire and imagination. If there is a zone where it is weakest, it is in the scientific and especially biochemical aspects. Nieper fills this gap, if necessary, single handed. His command of technical data is enormous. His mercurial intellect, near miraculous. Though still a young man, he must rank in the senior echelons of the new fight against cancer.

His own feeling is that cancers are of trophoblastic or embryonic nature. The question instantly arises, why do those over-functioning cells escape recognition and destruction by the body's own defences? It is already known that cells from tumours in tadpoles and mice, when cloned, give rise to normal tadpoles and mice. The genome of the malignant cells, that is the characteristic chromosomal make up, must thus be normal for the species rather than in some way mutant. Nieper meets this problem head on with the claim that there is a superimposed abnormality and that this probably manifests itself as a mucoid, shielding layer around the cell, which disguises it and prevents both recognition and attack.

The healthy body appears to have a way of 'clearing' cells for recognition, probably a 'tumosterone' similar to the prednisone group of adrenal compounds. Nieper suspects this tumosterone is derived from adrenal products, thymus gland products, vitamin D and light, of the kind that enters the eyes rather than falling on the skin.

Nieper's dedication is to the vital nature of aiding the de-shielding process. In his plan of cancer management there are three distinct phases though these may overlap. First the body is aided in its preparations to resist. Second, de-shielding is mandatory using such substances as heparin to break down the mucoid layer, as well as bromelanes (enzymes), beta-carotene, and zinc. Finally anti-cancer drugs like laetrile or its active breakdown component, benzaldehyde, are administered.

Another principle of Nieper's method is that as soon as a de-shielding agent ceases to function, malignant cells re-shield. Thus the attack must be continuous and prolonged. Careful adjustment of zinc and copper balances is important, as is lithium orotate. BCG is used in some circumstances as well as selenium, high vitamin C intake, and the use of gamma globulins.

Nieper's claims of vastly improved cure rates for many kinds of cancer are now being statistically surveyed. If the results are as he already believes, and there is no reason to doubt this, the breakthrough sought for so long and so in vain, in other ways, will be common knowledge.

He himself sums things up most succinctly[7]. "The old mechanistic approach (to cancer) is still done . . . but scientifically speaking it is hopelessly out of date."

*   *   *   *   *

Dr. Max Gerson died in 1959. But in the thirty years before his death he did perhaps more than any man had done before to explore the treatment of chronic diseases and to propose and practise new methods of management.

In the preface to his magnificent book *A Cancer Therapy*[8] he alludes, without bitterness, to the opposition his ideas had received. "The history of science, art and technique shows that each new idea has been fought bitterly; most of the reformers did not live to see the realization of their ideas." He understood that most doctors are cautious and unadventurous. That they attach too much devotion to what they see and to scientific proof, and too little to innovation. That they think what they have been taught is eternally right, and they they do not think at all what they have not been taught. That all innovation is left to a handful of others, deprives the profession and the world of much potential good.

Gerson faced this problem at a time when the alternative medicine movement was scarcely even born. Nevertheless he finally propounded what is now known as the Gerson Therapy. It is, as he claimed, a method that "usually produced dramatic initial improvements with chronic degenerative diseases within one week". The diseases he listed include cancer, migraine, multiple sclerosis, asthma, skin conditions, diabetes, allergies, heart disease, blood pressure and arthritis.

[7]Lecture at Royal Society of Medicine, London, 31 May 1980.
[8]Gerson, M., *A Cancer Therapy*. Totality Books, Del Mar, Calif., USA, 1958.

His method sought to overcome the century-long pessimism about cancer with an overwhelming optimism. Cancer was to be combatted by restoring function to the oxidising systems of the body, this being a theory developed from the knowledge that malignant cells thrive in a low-oxygen milieu. The three groups of his attack are (1) detoxification, (2) provision of essential minerals of the potassium group, and (3) giving oxidising enzymes largely derived from specially prepared nutritious drinks.

Gerson's therapy was a holistic form of treatment long before the name had been invented. He saw that the entire individual must be treated, not just one part. He stressed the value of diet similar to the Bio-Diet (see Chapter Seven). He savagely attacked salt for its dangers, and sought virtually to eliminate it. At a time when it must have sounded like heresy, he proclaimed that "ice cream is poison for children". He aimed, in his treatment, to decrease cellular content of sodium and replace it by potassium. He stressed the integral role of the liver in preventing and combatting cancer, and that support to liver function is therefore a basic tenet of cancer treatment.

Conversely he felt that the prospect of immunisation against cancer was not possible. At that time the existence of tissue specific anti-sera was not widely known. One cannot help feeling that had he lived long enough to learn of them, he might have changed his mind, and used them especially for liver protection and stimulation.

Gerson's actual programme is a complicated one. The patient's entire life must be built, for a while, around the treatment. As such it will also need the near full-time care of one or two attendants. The saltless diet is not easy to achieve and is unwelcome to many cancer patients, a large proportion of whom may have developed the disease in the first place because they are salt lovers.

The demands of the Gerson diet are very precise. Many things are forbidden, including sharp spices, alcohol, chocolate, refined sugar and flour, cream, cakes, nuts, mushrooms, soy, cucumber, pineapples and water. Preserved foods are similarly excluded, as are most fats and oils. Dairy produce is temporarily forbidden. Gerson gives the most detailed instructions for preparing vegetables and for making the nutritious drinks. Even the kind of grinder and juice extractor is special, as he felt that air contact with consequent exposure to oxygen, and even electro-magnetic influences taking place during preparations were relevant.

Other aspects of the treatment include a caffeine enema, up to six times a day, hourly special green or liver drinks, and supplements of potassium, iodine, thyroid gland, Royal Jelly, vitamins and enzymes.

However strange these ideas seem on first reading, there is little doubt that they work. The similarities of many of them with various components of the modern Gentle Method will be obvious enough. If there is one criticism to be offered, it is that Gerson's method is still being applied today with little alteration. Some feel that he would have changed it to accommodate newly arriving knowledge. Others defend the unchanged application of the method by saying that that is the Gerson Method, and that changes would make it something else.

Since his death, Gerson's work has been carried on by his daughter at a clinic devoted entirely to his specialised therapy. In addition to treating cancer, a far wider spectrum of diseases is being successfully managed, notably the disastrous demyelinating neurological conditions like multiple sclerosis. In Europe, Gerson's grand-daughter, Margaret Gerson Straus, conducts a powerful one-woman campaign from her home in London. Her lectures up and down the country are packed out. Her allotted time is always over-run as frantic chairmen try to conclude the barrages of questions that greet her. Her tireless energy and selfless devotion to the work and personality of the remarkable Max Gerson are something of which, there can be little doubt, the great man himself would thoroughly approve.

A final quote from Gerson is worth including.

> "For the future of coming generations, I think it is high time
> that we changed our agriculture and food preservation
> methods. Otherwise, we will have to increase our institutions
> for mental patients yearly, and we will see the hospitals
> overcrowded with degenerative diseases, even more rapidly
> and in greater numbers than the hospitals themselves can be
> enlarged."

Gerson wrote that a quarter of a century ago!

*   *   *   *   *

Dr. Peter Stephan is a homoeopathic practitioner working in London. He came to his present interest in cancer gradually and without any conscious attempt, simply because he found it to be occurring with increasing frequency in his other work.

Stephan's work in the last decade has been mostly concerned with the development of the field of Therapeutic Immunology, one of the two main aspects of the anti-ageing treatment known as Regenerative Therapy. (This latter is discussed in greater detail in Chapter Seven in view of its value as an adjunct to the Gentle Method.) In his work, which followed on from that begun in England by his father, Stephan makes wide use of the tissue specific antisera already mentioned as having been discovered by Dr. Jean Thomas, and recommended by Dr. Josef Issels over ten years ago[9]. His extensive research programmes have included one on the value of the sera in skin diseases, carried out in London, and another in the combat of arthritic conditions, carried out by the Huntingdon Research Centre.

But it is the value of this method in restraining the ravages of the age processes that interested Stephan most. His experience in this field in the United Kingdom is unequalled. It was through this interest in age that Stephan's concern with cancer grew. The increasing incidence of cancer with age is not only well documented, it is something that cannot fail to impress itself on the minds of those of us who work in either field.

Stephan brings a forthright freshness to the matter of cancer. Absent are the high-flown academic data and complex biochemical jargon. He sees the whole subject against a no-nonsense, common-sense background. Cancer, he declares, occurs in stressed tissues, and nowhere else. There are numerous ways in which different tissues can be sufficiently stressed. Chemical factors like alcohol stress the gastric mucosa and can cause stomach cancer. Tobacco smoke does the same to lungs. Sunlight does it to the skin. The breast tissues that have suffered from earlier mastitis are stressed. So is the uterine cervix that has been exposed to a multiplicity of different kinds of male sperm.

That is only half of the picture according to Stephan. For the stress factor, he feels, will not result in a 'successful' tumour growing unless the whole action takes place in a vulnerable body. For example, inadequate function of the reticulo-endothelial system may weaken resistance. So may hormone imbalance, by encouraging hormone dependent tumours when one or other hormone is present in unbalanced excess. Incorrect diet he also places high on his list of vulnerability factors.

The principle of using sera in cancer therapy is two-fold. First there is the curative programme in which affected tissues are challenged with the corresponding anti-serum, while at the same time, 'supportive' tissues like blood producing tissues, reticulo-endothelium, liver and so on, are stimulated by their specific equivalents. In this way the aim is to restrict the tumour and simultaneously promote defences. Perhaps even more important is the preventive aspect, for in this, as is the aim of all Regenerative Therapy, it is sought to pre-empt the onset of disease. Combination antisera are used of the tissues prone to high cancer incidence, breast, uterus, lung, colon, skin, and so on. By giving these in annually repeated, prophylactic courses, not only is cancer incidence reduced, but other problems of diminished functions of those areas that come with increasing age, are also substantially reduced.

Stephan feels he is on the verge of a huge breakthrough. It is still

[9] As ref. 6, see page 60.

in the late experimental stage, he says (in early 1981), yet when it is announced it will make all earlier methods, including those in previous Therapeutic Immunology, look like just so many packets of aspirins!

As hope springs eternal it is reasonable to have confidence in Stephan's ideas and enthusiasm. But whatever transpires, one thing is already certain. Both Stephan and I have been collecting and assessing the data of a large number of people who have undergone the anti-ageing influences of one or other kind of Regenerative Therapy over a period of years. Even preliminary figures are encouraging. For they suggest that overall, counting cases who have thorough and regular treatment courses, and those who have only occasional ones, there appears to be a reduction of over 11% in cancer coincidence per year. And for those who are thorough enough, this figure looks like being almost trebled! In combination with the rest of the Gentle Method programme, I believe we are already into a remarkable success story.

*   *   *   *   *

Dr. O. Carl Simonton is a physician specialising in the orthodox treatment of cancer by radiation. But he is now best known as leader of a very different approach to cancer therapy, that of visualisation.

Some ten years ago he wanted to arrange an experimental programme with patients at the University of Oregon. The aim was to try using two radiation treatments each day, instead of the usual one. To his surprise Simonton found patients to be unenthusiastic. On going into the reason he discovered that the patients lacked motivation. They didn't really think they could get well anyway, so the extra effort was not worth it to them.

At that stage Simonton began to seek other ways of stimulating motivation. He hit on the idea of teaching patients deep relaxation. Then, while they were relaxed, he asked them to visualise the radiation waves passing into the body and attacking the cancer cells. The initial success was encouraging. From here, together with Stephanie Simonton he developed and refined the technique. Others who learned also varied the method slightly in their own ways.

Now, basically, after learning relaxation, which is in itself a strongly beneficial technique, the patients are taught visualisation in detail. They are shown pictures and microscope slides of exactly what cancer cells and healthy cells look like. They may well examine their own X-ray pictures and, where available, study their own tissues removed during surgery, under high power magnification. Then, while relaxing, they visualise the 'good' active cells of the immune system attacking the diseased and despised cancer cells. In graphic terms they picture the helpful radiation waves and the molecules of chemotherapeutic drugs joining the attack. They see it all as a huge battle, with tumour cells succumbing and healthy cells growing back into the area, repairing damage, removing debris, restoring health.

So far there are no reliable facts and figures to show the effect of Simonton's work. It certainly generates hope; it certainly encourages a positive attitude of patient-involvement in therapy. These are bound to be advantageous factors. The Simontons believe cancer is one way in which people respond to stress. They see relaxation as a way of avoiding or compensating for stress. As such they regard it as having a value in preventing cancer, and in treating it.

The Simonton Visualisation Method has become very widely known in the United States, though far less well known elsewhere. In a leading article[10] the author quotes Wendy Schain, who counsels breast cancer patients for the National Cancer Institute, as saying that some forty per cent of her patients at least mention Simonton techniques and about half of these believe they can help in their particular case.

The Simontons are spreading their ideas by running training sessions for non-medical counsellors to learn visualisation before going out to teach and counsel patients. To British minds, their Research Centre in Fort Worth, Texas, and the rustic teaching camp an hour's drive away at Briarwood, would seem to be rather too carried away. Counsellors spend a lot of time deeply probing for repressed aggressions and anger, exploring feelings, deliberately emotional role-playing, and so on. "There is a lot of hugging and closeness and a lot of love," Simonton explains.

A pilot study of results shows that in patients with advanced malignancies, on average, patients lived twice as long as expected. This result, on the surface, is impressive. The problem is that the 'as long as expected' is a purely hypothetical estimate. What is more, the method attracts a certain quality of patient, even a kind of personality, the person determined to fight their disease. We have already seen that a fighting spirit has been proven to be associated with a longer life span anyway. Also, only patients who are well enough to travel to the Simontons and who can afford the treatment are included in the study, and this group is known to have a better life expectation anyway.

A danger of the Simonton method is one that it has in common with a number of other unorthodox methods practised by the unqualified. Its adherents easily become too enthusiastic. They are prone to regard the method as a strongly curative process, taking its values to too great an extreme and far more literally than does the inventor

[10]Kolata, G., *Smithsonian* (magazine of Smithsonian Institute, Washington), Vol. 11, No. 5, p. 49. August 1980.

himself.

Simonton sees his method as a highly beneficial part of overall orthodox therapy. In other words, he believes it should be used as an adjunct to treatment by surgery, radiation and chemotherapy. He does not claim it as a curative process that can stand alone and be effective unless combined with other techniques.

I share this view, but see no reason why it should not also be extended to be an adjunct of unorthodox methods. Indeed, I think that of the two it is more effective used that way.

To summarise, there is quite definite value in Simonton Visualis- ation Therapy. Not all of the thousands who have learned and used it can be wrong. My own opinion and experience convince me that all forms of relaxation are good in themselves as a form of deep resting. They are also valuable as routes to improved levels of suggestion, moral support, and the curtailment of depressions and despair. My own experience of visualisation, or imagery as it is sometimes called, supports the common sense view, that such adjuncts are bound to be helpful, but that they are best used as part of an integrated programme like the Gentle Method.

*　　*　　*　　*　　*

Frank Hourigan is not a doctor nor even a lay medical practitioner. In fact his own work is in unrelated scientific research. But as a one-man, walking compendium of knowledge of heterodox cancer therapy methods he is unequalled.

As the field of this kind of treatment expands, it repeatedly becomes noticeable that many ideas thought of as new are, in reality, merely more precise re-applications of old, even ancient principles. Hourigan's scouring of past literature has yielded vast amounts of useful data. What is more, applying his unique mixture of personal common sense, and no-nonsense, with his astute scientific acumen, the data, old and new, has enabled him to form valuable and perceptive theories of his own.

He is largely devoted to the Gerson Therapy as a fundamental principle, as are many of us. But he is gradually approaching the emergence of an overall pattern of cancer cause and treatment in which that is only a major part. As he sees it, heterodox therapies are now virtually able to offer a *cure* of cancer, rather than just a ridding of the body of cancerous cells. The shortcoming of the Gerson Therapy he regards as its failure to offer successful treatment to those who have severe liver damage, the similar exclusion of those who have had cobalt radiation, and its extreme dependence on the quality of equipment, fresh produce, and devoted human time. Conversely, he points out, a supremely logical attraction of the Gerson Therapy is that it was not, like orthodox methods, decided upon and evolved *in spite of* its effects on the patient. Rather, it was evolved "in the wake of clinical experience". Gerson's own quotation, "The result at the sick bed is decisive", he says, is far more logical than persisting in a method that hopes (but fails) to prove a theory. Few could disagree with this.

Hourigan constantly reminds of the valued work of the past. For example, the use in the fifties[11] of a combination of zinc, magnesium and vitamin C given by intravenous injection at frequent intervals. A clinical trial on over 200 cases yielded results so remarkable that one can only wonder why it was not followed up avidly by other workers. But he also turns his eyes towards the future, foreseeing the use of pulsed magnetic fields (PMF) to cancer therapy. Already there is published work to show the use of PMF in healing, malunited bone fractures and restoration of part-severed spinal cords in experimental animals. Hourigan believes that application of PMF to the diseased liver of cancer patients is an area of much potential growth.

Looking backwards again, he draws attention to the mixed toxin 'vaccine' composed of bacterial fragments used before World War One, and known as Coley's Fluid. This produced deliberate inflammation in tissues surrounding the growth. In his time Coley was much honoured. In fact his work was duplicated, an accepted indication of the accuracy of his tests and reports. But with the arrival of antibiotics and the reduction of interest in the therapeutic applications of immunology his work dropped out of fashion. This is strange if the published figures of 50% success in treatment of the bone tumour, osteogenic sarcoma, are anything like accurate. For orthodox treatment of amputation with or without radiation, and chemotherapy, is a 70% failure, yet is retained as a treatment.

Perhaps Hourigan explains things when, writing of this very point[12] he says, "An even better touchstone to the effectiveness of Coley's technique is provided by the American Cancer Society, who placed 'Coley's Fluid' upon their list of quack remedies. With their track record this amounts to an accolade."

Hourigan keeps extensive records of cases he hears about or sees, either personally, or in new as well as old literature. From this mass of data, and the thought that goes into accumulating and considering it, he propounds a number of his own, or revised guidelines. At other times he puts a whole concept into a sentence or two. One cannot do better than simply to quote him with minimum explanatory comment.

[11] Meyer, and others.
[12] Hourigan, F., Personal communication to author.

(Speaking of the way unexpected degrees of response may well result from some aspect of treatment), "The metabolic therapist should always be ready to take action to change the main thrust of the therapy to take advantage of such happy accidents."

"If a rising dose of pancreatic enzyme is being taken, any 'sick headache' or 'I feel awful' symptom should be regarded with suspicion. If it clears with great rapidity after a coffee enema, then builds up again, the dose should be stopped as a check."

(Speaking of the way metabolic therapy can cause destruction of malignant tissue), "The great problem with the approach is that the permissible rate of destruction of the malignant tissue (and thus the rate of application of the therapy) must be governed by the ability of the liver to detoxify the resulting products."

"The effective single dose of (enzyme) chymotrypsin on the average advanced cancer patient is of the order of 15 g, due to the necessity of offsetting the level of tumour-protecting chymotrypsin inhibitor entering the bloodstream from the malignant tissue."

"The well-supported detoxifying liver can remove the antagonist (tumour-protecting inhibitor) from the blood stream."

"It was a tragedy that this medical genius [Gerson] was ignored in his lifetime. It would be an equal tragedy if, because he left a book on his therapy, this were regarded as unchangeable holy writ of which we may alter no jot."

"I recall a case where 18 g of ascorbic acid per day (in a 75 kg patient) was needed to prevent scurvy symptoms caused by immature white cells scavenging vitamin C from the serum. It is almost impossible to saturate the system (with vitamin C) in advanced cases."

"The administration of amygdalin (B17) in the early stages of classical Gerson Therapy can be fatal" (as further malignant tissue destruction may result, and may overload a hard-pressed liver).

"Cameron and Pauling quote only 9-10% of long term recoveries in their (metabolically treated) cases. But the total proportion of patients who obtain partial relief is considerably larger."

And finally, a pearl of what is at the same time advice and encouragement. Discussing the way that some components of Gentle Method treatments appear to have several different beneficial effects . . . "Nature never uses stools with one leg."

This latter points out a common pitfall of 'scientific medicine' . . . that of regarding specific and single phenomena as having only single and specific causes. Things are never that simple, or precisely compartmented. As has been wisely said before, Nature abhors boundaries and shades off her dividing lines. Frank Hourigan, it seems, recognises no boundaries anyway!

*   *   *   *   *

The cases now to be described were chosen by me on a purely arbitrary basis. They were not selected to show how good or how bad one or other method of cancer treatment might be. Rather, they were chosen because each, in some way, is instructive in pointing out dangers or pitfalls. A long series of cases all making more or less the same critical or complimentary points, I think, would be worthless.

Neither, I should add, are any of these cases my own. In one or two instances I have known or briefly advised either the patient or the medical attendant, but only by virtue of being consulted. None of the cases has been at any time under my supervision. I report them dispassionately therefore, claiming no credit and shouldering no blame.

The main value of including such story-like case histories is that undoubtedly people identify more with real instances that have actually happened to folk like themselves, than they do with tables of statistics. What is more, medical statistics are made of real people, something that is easily overlooked.

*   *   *   *   *

Marion D. was just thirty-six years old when, in May 1976, she attended her family planning clinic for a routine cervical smear. She had always had satisfactory general health, had had an illegitimate pregnancy in her teens, and had been on an oral contraceptive pill for about six years. She was a heavy smoker at 30-35 cigarettes a day.

She was both shocked and horrified when her smear report was positive, showing that she had very early malignant changes (known as carcinoma in situ).

Three weeks later she entered the West London Hospital for a cone biopsy. This involves taking a cone-shaped piece out of the neck of the uterus. The aim is not primarily to remove the growth, it is to provide a specimen for thorough microscopic examination. If most or all the malignancy is also removed that is regarded as an added advantage.

The report on Marion's biopsy was discouraging. It showed dysplasia, the kind of growth recognised as pre-cancerous, and it also showed more actual carcinoma. The pathologist further commented that it was not possible to say whether the tumour had been completely removed or not, as the affected area went right to the edge of the specimen. Followed up three weeks later it was reported that the cervix had healed. No further arrangements were made beyond planning a further smear for four months later.

Particularly important was the fact that this patient was now allowed to depart from close medical supervision without any advice as to what she could do to improve her chances of recovery. She was merely to remain under periodic observation.

In February 1977, at further examination, the cervix was again found to be inflamed and a small polyp was discovered. If a repeat smear was done it was mislaid, for it does not appear in her hospital records (which I have before me as I write). Six months later the cervix was still inflamed and eroded. In March 1978 another smear was taken. This time it survived. It was abnormal. Two months later it was decided to do a very thorough visual examination of the cervix, and because of its appearance at that stage, another more extensive biopsy was taken.

The report was the worst so far. It showed that the patient by that time already had an infiltrating carcinoma of the squamous type. In everyday language this means that a serious degree of malignancy had been reached in the neck of the uterus. The only possible orthodox recommendation was complete removal and the patient was advised to undergo hysterectomy forthwith.

It was at this point that she decided she did not want to lose her uterus. In spite of being in her late thirties, she had not totally abandoned the idea of further motherhood. What is more, she felt that loss of this organ would reduce her feeling of feminity. For these and other reasons she therefore sought the aid of unorthodox medicine.

She came under the care of a London homoeopath who has already been discussed in this chapter. He gave advice on diet, lifestyle, her disastrous smoking habits, her exercise programme and her intake of vitamins and minerals. After routine laboratory examination of her blood and urine biochemistry showed no other serious abnormality, he devised for her a complex programme of anti-sera, mainly of reticulo-endothelial and genital tissues but also of the organs of detoxification and waste elimination. The patient's consultant was informed and, to his credit, although he was unhappy about it, he neither disapproved nor forbad the therapy.

Three months later when she returned to her consultant he was, to his admitted surprise, obliged to report that both her latest cervical smear and her vaginal examination was entirely normal. He has continued to do routine check-ups on her ever since. When last spoken to (January 1981), she remained fit and well without further treatment or gynaecological symptoms of any kind.

This case teaches several lessons. First, that orthodox doctors can consent to unorthodox therapies for their patients, that turn out to be beneficial. Second, that anti-serum therapy can effectively treat cancer, and not merely abate it, leaving it prone to early recurrence when treatment stops. Third, and most important of all, it shows the danger of merely keeping a case of cancer under observation.   Marion D.'s malignancy did in fact recur. She should have been on strong counter therapies from the very start. No case of cancer exists in which it is safe simply to keep a watch for recurrence. A full anti-cancer regime is mandatory, and unless he orders it, the attending physician is guilty of neglect.

*   *   *   *   *

Fiona N. first found a lump in her right breast on a routine check that she carried out every month. That was in the summer of 1978. She was 45 years old, a busy housewife who also helped run her husband's business, doing both jobs with a seemingly inexhaustible supply of energy. She saw her family doctor two days later and was told of his suspicions that the lump might well be malignant.

Within two weeks the lump was removed and examined and the diagnosis was confirmed. Mastectomy was performed after two further weeks and several enlarged glands were removed from the axilla. All were involved, showing that the malignancy had already metastasised.

Whole body examination (scan) revealed no other suspect areas. A course of radiotherapy was carried out six weeks later. There was extensive burning of the chest wall and the surgical wound broke down for a length of four inches. The patient's condition deteriorated and she became very ill for the first time she could remember. There was a great degree of nausea, loss of appetite and weight loss. After a period of rest and recuperation the patient entered hospital for chemotherapy.

There was again a substantial loss of weight. The patient lost all her hair and became emotionally distressed. She relinquished all her few remaining commitments to her home and the business.

For seven months she began to show some improvement. The chest wound healed slowly and she was relieved by the departure of the offensive smell it had generated. She then began gradually to get symptoms of alternating episodes of constipation and diarrhoea. Abdominal examination showed the presence of fluid (ascites). Her liver was slightly enlarged, and the surgeon thought that smaller masses, probably swollen lymph glands, could be felt deeper in the abdomen.

Fluid drawn from the abdominal cavity by paracentesis, contained malignant cells. It was decided that the now multiple tumours were probably oestrogen influenced, so it was proposed to remove both ovaries, thus stopping oestrogen production. The operation was carried out in the summer of 1979.

There was a further period of slight improvement before she began to deteriorate again. Another course of chemotherapy was carried out, producing even more marked deterioration, and at one point she was in and out of a coma for almost a week. After a measure of recovery, the collection of abdominal fluid recurred and became so severe that she had to have the abdominal contents tapped off every two weeks. The next surgical opinion was that removal of the pituitary gland from the skull may yet further delay the worsening of symptoms. She underwent cranial surgery in the spring of 1980.

Fiona N. is not a patient of mine, but I do know her. She is now a small, shrunken, pathetic creature. Her vitality and personality have ebbed to nothing, though she remains adamant about her intention to fight on. She has been told that no more treatment is possible. She awaits her doom with commendable fortitude, regretting only the effect that her ordeal has had on her husband and two sons. I believe she will not survive to see this volume published.

This case teaches three all too familiar lessons. First, that the treatment has been excessive and appalling in its effect on the patient and her family. Second, that it has been utterly fruitless, in that she will surely die. I personally believe she would have lived at least as long without treatment, and that most important of all, she would probably have enjoyed her last two or three years far more if she had been left alone. She had all the intelligence, character and fortitude to have done just that.

Finally, and this is unforgivable, throughout her entire therapy programme, she has not once received any supportive anti-cancer treatment. No advice about diet, no vitamins, no extra supplements of any kind. This is the kind of medical malpraxis I have discussed elsewhere.

*   *   *   *   *

Alec F. and Alec C. do not know each other. They share the same name, both are aged 54 and both are the owners of small provincial garages. Both became ill in the spring of 1980 with symptoms of abdominal pain, episodes of vomiting and a feeling of being generally not well. Both sought the advice of family doctors and were referred to hospital for surgical opinion. In both instances a diagnosis of cancer of the large bowel was made and in both cases it was found that the liver was involved in a fairly advanced malignant spread.

Their cases were not uncommon. Neither was the advice they were given. The orthodox routine suggested in each case was that surgery (colostomy) was necessary to remove the bowel tumour and prevent the blockage thought to be imminent in each of them. Surgery was to be followed by a chemotherapy regime.

Alec C. accepted his doctor's advice. Colostomy was performed, about half of his colon being removed. The severed end was brought out through a hole in the abdominal wall (a stoma) so that his faeces could be voided into a neat, disposable polythene bag that he wore under his clothing. In only a short time he claimed he had become accustomed to the slight odour that came from it. It was unfortunate that his wife remained very sensitive to the odour. They therefore moved to separate bedrooms. The emotional state was complicated further in that she felt unable to have sexual relations with him, partly because of the smell and partly because of the repellent nature of his apparatus.

Six weeks after the operation he underwent prolonged chemotherapy with the usual result of hair loss, weight loss and profound ill health. He handed his business over to a manager who ruined it within six months. At that stage the patient took over again but has not had the stamina to rebuild it. His wife has since established a relationship with another man (an old family friend).

The patient's treatment prevented the anticipated obstruction, but has in other respects proved unsuccessful. He has not been able to regain his health, forfeited during the chemotherapy. His liver infiltration is worse. The last year has been one of painful surgery, worsening symptoms added to by those resulting from chemotherapy, social, domestic and financial stress. At his last assessment, after being advised that there was no further worthwhile treatment, he demanded to know his estimated expectation of life. His doctors were reluctant to tell him but finally stated that he could expect a further six months.

Alec F. had one small advantage over his unknown fellow sufferer. His doctor told him the truth about the seriousness of his diagnosis. He also told him surgery would relieve the blockage but that the further outlook was hopeless. Treatment, he stated, could be expected to postpone death but that twelve to eighteen months was the likely duration of his life. He also, in reply to close questioning, told his patient exactly what the treatment would involve in terms of pain, other symptoms and the problems of colostomy.

The doctor advised his patient to start on treatment at once. The patient declined and within three weeks had located a practitioner who started him off on a full Gentle Method routine. Within a week the abdominal pains ceased. The patient lost 15 lb in weight, but had been about that much overweight to start with. During the second week he had his last attack of vomiting. This he ascribed to trying to take too many liver drinks. Over the course of four weeks he improved to the point of declaring to his doctor that he felt better than he had for years.

He was fortunate in that, although he did not think the patient was doing the right thing, the doctor continued to supervise his treatment. Indeed, he seized the opportunity to experience the Gentle Method alternative at first hand and for the first time.

Alec F.'s condition has remained almost unaltered for nearly a year now. There has been no return of bowel obstruction symptoms. He has declined check x-rays to see how his bowel tumour is progressing. But liver scan shows no change. The liver involvement has not decreased. What is surprising the doctor is that it has not got greater. That, and the fact that the patient is in better general health than the doctor has ever known him in. He is hard at work, and apart from bringing his will up to date his illness has caused him no problems, he says.

It is not possible at this stage to estimate how long Alec F. has to live. He may, like Alec C., be within six months of his death. Having seen both cases, I doubt this. He looks good for years.

But it is worthless making opinionated guesses at the outcome. What is not so useless is to compare the last eighteen months of life of these two men. If both are to succumb this year, which, I offer for judgement, has had the better time of things? Orthodox treatment has, at great cost, done nothing apparent to change the course of Alec C.'s disease. Unorthodox treatment may or may not have put years on Alec F.'s life but it has unquestionably put more life in his years.

*   *   *   *   *

Harry D., at the age of 36, was already a senior partner in a prominent company of solicitors just outside London when his real problems began. He would fit, in many ways, the traditional description of the perfect English gentleman. Above average height, blonde, superbly proportioned, weighing in at 210 lbs, with a dry sense of humour and immaculate, quiet, good manners.

For years he had had a small dark mole on the skin of his back exactly in the mid-line between his shoulder blades. He went on holiday to Africa with his wife and two small children. The weather was superb and they all spent almost a month swimming, playing on the beach and basking in the endless warm sunshine.

Six weeks after their return he noticed that his mole was inclined to itch, something it had never done before. As he couldn't see it, his wife checked and thought it looked no different apart from perhaps being a bit larger. They thought nothing more of it, but the itching persisted and got worse. He could not reach it to scratch, so there had to be some other explanation when, a month or so later, he found blood on his pyjama jacket one morning. On re-examination, his wife reported that the mole had doubled in size since she'd last looked at it.

Harry's doctor told him point blank that he thought the mole had become malignant. Three days later the mole was removed for examination. It took an inexplicable (and unforgivable) three weeks for the report to become available. The diagnosis was a melanoma, a tumour recognised as being of very high grade malignancy. The patient was re-admitted to hospital and the entire surrounding area of the mole was widely excised. As the exposed area was so extensive and could be expected to heal only slowly, the wound was closed by a skin graft taken from his thigh. Both the graft and the donor area became grossly infected. High doses of antibiotics failed to control the infection and the wounds broke down.

The infected areas were carefully cleaned and dressed daily and after several weeks they eventually healed.

The patient received no further treatment, no dietary supplements, and no further medical supervision was recommended. (He was being treated not under the National Health Service, but privately.) He remained very fit and well, and after about sixteen months the entire incident was half forgotten when one day he leaned across a desk and in so doing noticed a small tender lump on the sternum (breast-bone). His doctor, anxious at the new discovery, had the lump removed. Harry's tumour had reappeared.

There was worse news to come. A full body scan was carried out in view of the remoteness of the second tumour from the first. Multiple other masses were located in both lungs, the abdomen and inside the skull. Immediate treatment involved direct radiation to the head. There was extensive burning, total hair loss and marked personality changes. Chemotherapy was given by intravenous drip. The patient lost 60 lb in less than four weeks. His children became afraid of his altered appearance and mannerisms, and he felt he had to stop cuddling them or entering their rooms. He became morose, for a short while suicidal, and sexually impotent.

Repeated body scan after eight weeks showed no change in the size of the various tumours. Showing immense courage he agreed to undergo a further series of thirty more exposures to radiation, mostly of his head and lungs, and these were explained to him as life-saving and extending measures. When just over halfway through the course, he expressed the opinion that he no longer regarded the kind of life he was having as justifying the horror of trying to extend it. He was hospitalised for the rest of the course, mainly to reduce the very real and recognised risk of suicide.

He survived the therapy and was discharged. Further scan two weeks before the writing of this report (January 1981) revealed that there had been no response to treatment.

In desperation this very orthodox gentleman agreed to accept some measure of unorthodox medication for the first time. He has just started on the only things he will take, megavitamins by mouth, and injections and tissue-specific antisera of lung, cerebral cortex, stomach, and lymphatic and reticulo-endothelial systems, given in suppository form.

I believe it is too little and too late. His immune response capability is likely to be virtually nil. I believe his family will spend next Christmas without him. Yet again, it is a particularly tragic waste.

Harry D.'s case also yields several lessons. First, it is a mistake to think cancer is a disease of weak, old people. He was apparently healthy and far from old. Second, the danger of strong sunlight, especially to fair people. I have no doubt that the unaccustomed exposure was a major factor in initiating malignant change. Third, there is the ever-present medical hazard of regarding check-ups as the same thing as prevention, . . . only in this case the patient did not even receive these check-ups. Constant vigilance is imperative after a diagnosis of cancer. Fourth, this must surely be an extreme example of the worthless horror of this kind of therapy. To perpetrate such monstrous techniques unless there is a substantial expectation of cure is callous, misguided, and should be forbidden by law if it cannot be curtailed by moral obligation.

Finally, it is worth remembering, once more, that Harry D., like countless others, was allowed to pass out of medical supervision without the least attempt to impose an anti-cancer support regime or even helpful dietary supplements.

Had it not been for this culpable neglect, his family would, I believe, have had a better time next Christmas.

*   *   *   *   *

Dr. Naomi S. was in her middle forties when she found her breast lump. She rightly suspected the worst, took a day off from her medical practice and had the lump removed for examination. Her colleague, a pathologist whom she knew, confirmed the diagnosis of carcinoma.

In order that there should be no local discussion in the village in which she worked, she went immediately to the surgeon who is perhaps the most eminent in London in the field of breast surgery. Without hesitation he advised operation and follow up treatment with radiotherapy then possible subsequent chemotherapy. The arrangements for managing her practice were made, the doctor entered hospital and her diseased breast was removed.

The surgeon felt that surgery had been very successful, there having been no sign of spread beyond the breast and no evidence of involved lymph glands. It was consequently decided that there was no indication for chemotherapy, but that a course of post-operative radiotherapy would be a wise precaution. This was carried out over a period of a month and the patient returned home.

Dr. S. is a woman of considerable physical stature, of powerful personality and of most determined spirit. Additionally she is possessed of enormous energy, being both busy country doctor, housewife, and commander-in-chief of a big home in a large acreage of land, which latter she gardens to immaculate standards with only intermittent help. Her radiotherapy produced the anticipated period of general malaise, some weight loss, fatigue and emotional depression. However, her surgical wound healed well and quickly, and within a few weeks she had resumed full control of her home (which she never fully relinquished anyway) and had returned to full time medical practice.

This patient would have no sympathy whatsoever with any aspect of Alternative Medicine. Though thoroughly open-minded, she is of traditional training and experience and sees no advantage in departing from principles with which she is familiar. She has adhered to her usual gourmet diet (she is a cordon bleu cook), which is full of meats, creams and rich delicacies. She does not smoke, and drinks only the occasional sherry or table wine. About her one advantage, according to Gentle Method principles, is a liberal supply of fresh fruit and vegetables from her own garden . . . though these are usually cooked with butter or other deprecated ingredients. She takes no enzymes, no minerals and no vitamin supplements, remaining totally convinced that she can obtain all that is needed from her diet.

In spite of this total lack of supportive therapy, through the three years since her operation she has been regularly checked by her very fine surgeon. There has not been the remotest sign of recurrence. Dr. S. remains fit and well as ever, and just as hectically involved in her numerous exacting duties.

The writer has little doubt that this kind of courageous and determined fighter can beat cancer . . . it is, after all, in many ways, a *beaten disease* . . . and with only the weapons of orthodoxy. That being said, Dr. S. is exactly the calibre to win such a battle.

My only comment is that I would feel happier and would see it as good medical sense to add the extra in-depth layers of protection that would stem from use of unorthodoxy as well. There seems no point in not using the maximum number of safety precautions.

The doctor herself makes no comment about that at all. Apart from check-ups of diminishing frequency she regards the episode as virtually over. With unfailing sense of humour she states that the only difference the whole thing has meant to her is that sometimes, now, her husband "doesn't know what to do with his other hand".

It just shows that we too must keep an open mind. Orthodoxy *can* do it too . . . sometimes.

*   *   *   *   *

Mrs. Penny Brohn already had a wide experience of several aspects of Alternative Medicine when she suddenly found herself cast in the role of patient instead of practitioner. She is a highly skilled acupuncturist of several years standing who practises in the city of Bath. Her own training includes a university degree in Sociology, as well as a year in China studying under a medical acupuncturist who was himself the latest of sixteen generations of acupuncturists in his family. Her ability and integrity are above question. She is well known not only within her practice, but for her lectures and radio appearances on this and allied subjects.

She was thirty-six years old when she discovered a small, tender lump in her left breast. The lump, about an inch long, had the suspiciously typical feel, when examined by her doctor, of a possible malignancy. Removal of the lump for microscopy was recommended, but the authorities declined to permit acupuncture to be used as an anaesthetic.

Immediately after the discovery, the patient put herself on a homoeopathic remedy, specific for breast disease, called Phytolacca. She also received acupuncture from a colleague. She recalled two severe urinary infections during the previous year. She had also lost both her parents totally unexpectedly within two months of each other just a year or so before. She relates both of these episodes to the onset of her cancer. She had always been sensitive to hormone variations, being subject to pre-menstrual symptoms both before and after the birth of her three children.

The surgery conducted for her lump turned out to be complicated by considerable haemorrhage and massive generalised bruising afterwards. Microscopy confirmed the diagnosis of a breast carcinoma. She was advised to undergo immediate mastectomy, followed by radiation and possible subsequent chemotherapy. Her refusal to agree to this kind of treatment led at first to dismay and anxiety by those who were attending her, as well as from some members of her family. She declares quite firmly now, that not only was she advised, but pressured, towards the treatment. To some extent she agrees this was intended for her own good, though she feels that unnecessarily aggressive attitudes were adopted towards her. Finally her consultant assured her he thought that she would probably be alright for a month, he was doubtful about a second month, but that within three months she would be "in real trouble". That was in September 1979.

With the devoted help of her engineer husband, she sought alternative care but did not know where to find it. Later in the month she flew to Bavaria to the clinic of Dr. Josef Issels. She was aware, at that time, of feeling very ill indeed and she had serious doubts about her ability to survive.

She spent nine weeks under Issels' care, having immunotherapy enzymes, potassium and mineral supplements, HOT, negative ionisation and high frequency thymus and pituitary stimulation. As is often the case, the immunotherapy produced tenderness in her ovaries and in the right armpit, leading Issels to diagnose early involvement or pre-cancerous states in those areas too. After making only very slow progress to start, she began to improve and on leaving Germany she felt much better. Back at home she continued the therapy but also went onto a vegetarian diet. She also trained in biofeedback under Maxwell Cade, learning to influence both physical and mental processes. When she found a source of amygdalin she started oral dosage, and was surprised to find that there was a 'flare up' of the tenderness at the site of the original lump. She fortunately ascribed this to a favourable reaction, which it is, and persevered. After a few days the reaction subsided and amygdalin dosage has been continued at one gram daily without further side-effects.

Mrs. Brohn now feels that her 'brush with cancer' did her a great deal of good. Having, as she felt, stared death in the face, has given her, she believes, a new ability to confront the harder tasks of her life. She has become more disciplined, more resilient, more self-confident. Her relationship with her husband she describes as having matured more in a few weeks than it had in a decade of marriage, and more than it might have done ever without such a stimulus.

She considers that she met with much selfishness from some of the orthodox people with whom she came in contact, and whom, only half in jest, she now describes as the 'flat earth theorists'. She regards these people as having been hurt by her decision to decline orthodox treatments, sometimes offended, and often frightened, because what they believed might be proved wrong after all. Some, she goes as far as to say, would almost like to see her get worse, to be able to console themselves and to be able to say 'I told you so' because their own rightness and security means more to them, at a fundamental level, than does the welfare of the patient. It is understandable, she explains, for they have a lot to lose.

It is the abused person, the person of low self-image, who gets cancer, she thinks. The emotional catharsis of her period of illness she rates as having been of the highest benefit of all. She acquired the initiative to sort out her life. Now she regards herself as having a quality of life that is so great, that the question of whether or when her cancer is or will be cured is simply not the important factor. She is able to say, because of all this, 'Thank God I had cancer'.

Her cancer has totally disappeared and has shown no trace of recurrence in spite of the absence of the recommended orthodox therapy, and although she is now far into her second year of 'borrowed time'.

Mrs. Brohn is a truly remarkable lady who is, by virtue of her example and courage, a credit to herself and to her loved ones. She will, I am sure, go on to do great good, in both her professional and personal life, for many years.

CHAPTER SIX

THE GENTLE METHOD . . . THE PRINCIPLES

Steadily growing disillusionment with the form of cancer therapy and its low success rates provided the spur that initiated the equally steadily growing interest in alternative methods of the last two decades. Once again it was an example of sheer necessity being the mother of much delayed invention.

Now that things are on the move, it is becoming difficult for people to realise how hard it was to make progress in earlier days. Prominent thinkers and intrepid leaders like those mentioned in the previous chapter had already begun their work. The task must have appeared daunting. They faced the enormous edifice of solid professional opinion. Nothing of note had ever questioned either it or the medical people who managed it.

The medical establishment is hard to describe or even accept as a concept. But it exists. It does not live in one place, or society or group, though there are prominent organs where its power is displayed. Nonetheless it exists in almost every doctor's mind. He knows he is a member of a privileged elite. His income is secure, his status ensured. He will be protected by this formless but strong surrounding quality . . . as long as he remains a member. Providing he accepts the rules and performs within the permitted lattitudes he is safe. To step beyond the limits is to risk personal, professional and financial ruin.

This 'establishment' still exists and is very powerful even today. In many ways it is a good thing. The standards set, on the whole maintain a high professional integrity, and this, in turn, protects that vulnerable class of people, the patients. But it also resists change in many ways. The changing moral climate is just one example. In theory at least it is still possible for a doctor to lose his livelihood as a result of a physical indiscretion of extra-marital nature. Furthermore, a doctor tried and punished for a legal offence is one of the few people who could still face a further trial, by his professional peers, even after his debt to the community had been settled.

It is no part of this volume to discuss in detail the pros and cons of that state of affairs. Only in relation to cancer and its treatment is it relevant here. The point to be made is that the status quo of medicine, far from acting for the general good of cancer sufferers, actually militates against them. That is wholly bad. For a doctor to hold views that differed from the 'accepted' was risky. To speak up was even harder. To obtain research funds would be impossible.

The power of the establishment was suggested and exploited by subtle fund sources. Medical publications that could hardly be understood by any but doctors, fostered the atmosphere of 'them and us'. And these publications in turn were supported by the profits from advertising for drugs, medical equipment and so on. At a time when medical prestige and aura were being eroded by the patent shortcomings that result from socialised health services, the doctor's personal view of himself was being artifically supported by these means.

The result was that although more and more people, patients and doctors alike, were getting dissatisfied, little of this appeared on the surface, and nothing was done to improve matters.

At the same time a whole new movement was afoot. People were taking an interest in themselves, their bodies, and healthy living standards. Also at the same time, and as part of the same deep social upheaval, flower-power reached the streets, anti-war demonstrations shook governments, religious foundations lost adherents, and the health food crazes began. People began to read, learn, and think about themselves, the environment, the trends of commercial exploitation and so on.

Cracks appeared in the protective plating of long-reigning institutions. It was that way in alternative medicine. In private, doctors began to doubt and question and discuss. Occasional outbursts appeared in the press, mostly with resulting howls of derision. But gradually the ideas spread. Doctors even began meeting with and co-operating with 'unqualified' (in the sense of having no medical degrees) people like naturopaths and healers. Little progress seemed to take place for several years. In some quarters there was a detectable air of despondency.

Then suddenly everything took off. Nothing is as irresistable as an idea whose time has come. The movement is a bit like the launch of a space rocket. Lift off has happened but movement in the initial stages still appears unbelievably slow and precarious. The point is that full power has been applied. From now on everything will accelerate. New work is being done. Conferences are being held. Everywhere fresh, capable minds are turning, a bit reluctantly and with surprise to start, to ideas they had previously thought ridiculous, or more often, not thought about at all. Soon now, new ideas and concepts will emerge. New programmes will be launched. Gradually the entire emphasis of cancer treatment will alter.

But all this will take some time. It involves big changes and it will still meet with much resistance. In that time, a lot of people will die, and more still will suffer. There is no need, for the new ways to treat cancer are already with us and capable of use. Improvements galore are on the way, but there is no reason to await their arrival.

This chapter will explain the rationale, where it is known, of the new ideas. The next will tabulate both preventive and therapeutic programmes.

Using the contents of this book, the combined work of many people, cancer incidence can be cut by a huge proportion, and cancer death and suffering can be at least halved right now. There is no more need to wait.

* * * * *

The widespread occurrence of cancer and the huge numbers of sufferers, currently estimated at around six million deaths a year[1] has opened up an enormous commercial opportunity. There is, of course, no reason why disease and its care and cure should not attract a fee for those involved. What is sad is that such a dreadful disease should have undergone such a heinous exploitation. Cancer patients face near certain death. They are thus more vulnerable than most people. And they and their loved ones will consequently go to the most extreme lengths.

People being vulnerable, and others being greedy, comprises a one-sided economic situation in which cheating, lying and grasping have always flourished. Medical personnel are no different from anyone else in this characteristic. This has become painfully apparent from the recent professional corruption that has led to the American Medicare Scheme being investigated by the FBI, in what has become known as the Medifraud Scandal. Fraud by doctors, nursing homes and laboratories, especially in the form of kickbacks or commission-rate bribes, have cost the scheme billions of dollars. At one point over seven hundred serious cases were being investigated, mostly of unnecessary surgery and pathology tests being carried out. A top FBI official[2] declared, "Corruption has permeated virtually all of the Medicare and Medicaid health care industry."

[1] Peper, R.C., Chairman of (USA) House Select Committee on Ageing, *Frontiers of Cancer Research*, 1979.
[2] Mullen, F., Report to House of Representatives Committee, 1980.

I have no doubt that medical corruption also goes on on both sides, orthodox and unorthodox, of cancer care. This is not surprising as, in the 'cancer industry' more people appear to live partly or totally off the proceeds of cancer, than actually die from it. I have seen quite enough to know of what I write.

Lamentable though this all is in itself, it has another serious aspect, which has been seen in the hotly disputed laetrile controversy. Up to now laetrile has been a cornerstone of alternative cancer treatment methods. On one side the proponents of the substance have promoted it, often unscrupulously for the immense financial gain. Exaggerated and anecdotal reports put out by the hirelings of commercial enterprises posing as academic organisations have flooded the 'health press'. The other, establishment side, has unfairly cheated by conducting deliberately misleading trials of laetrile which were rigged to demonstrate its failure and so preserve their own status of superiority. The battle has become the important thing. The value of laetrile has become secondary. The controversy has overshadowed the facts and has prevented or postponed properly conducted research.

As laetrile is important it is as well to devote some further space to it. Laetrile, also known as vitamin B17, is the product of the plant *Prunus amygdalus*, the bitter almond plant. It is also found in a number of other plants of this type and is in high concentration in the pips (in USA called pits), the soft kernel found within the stone of peaches, cherries, almonds, and so on.

Pharmacologically it is known as amygdalin. Chemically it is a glycoside and it is a contraction, using only the first and last syllables of its more accurate chemical name, laevo-mandelo-nitrile, that forms the common name laetrile. The two opposing opinions are that it is new, dangerous, and useless, or that it is old, safe and effective. It is most certainly not new. Amygdalin has been known, written about and included in the pharmacopoea of several European countries for at least a century.

Originally it was postulated that amygdalin, once absorbed, is broken down into components like benzaldehyde, benzoic acid, thiocyanates and the all-important cyanide group. Certainly such breakdown products do result. It was then, probably wrongly, asserted that the cyanide material, which is so highly poisonous, is quickly eliminated from areas where it can do any harm, but remains in tumour tissues. This was said to be because the necessary enzymes to break down cyanide existed less in tumours, another very doubtful claim.

Such unsupported and unsupportable theories were quickly demolished by knowledgeable biochemists. There then followed a totally false deduction. This was that because the explanation was wrong, amygdalin was ineffective. This is not the case. A curious pseudoscientific examination of the effects of amygdalin was then carried out. A large number of doctors (reported as 385,000) were written to by an investigating doctor[3]. When a preponderance of replies unfavourable to amydgdalin were, as could be anticipated, received, it was held that this proved the inefficiency of the substance. That is nonsense, just as bad as the distorted biochemistry theory.

I suspect that new trials, now being initiated, will bear out the experience of physicians who, like myself, have used amygdalin for some years. I do not know the details of the biochemistry, though I think we shall find it is the benzaldehyde that is the effective de-shielding component of amygdalin. Like most physicians, I must be content to leave the biochemistry to those who are skilled in it, in the hope that they will be honest. But as a clinician, I claim a modest expertise. What I do know about is treating people with illnesses. And, in using amygdalin in the treatment of cancer, I have no doubt that it is markedly, not dramatically but markedly, helpful. It is an important part of sensible cancer treatment and must continue to be used unless and until superseded. Correctly administered, mostly by injection, it is entirely safe. It is, however, its concentration at the malignant tissue that matters. This must be kept high and continuously so, to be of maximum benefit. As it is quickly excreted, considerable amounts must be used. In general, I find, as with a number of other medical preparations, naturally extracted amygdalin is more effective than the pure, synthesised variety.

Failure of amygdalin therapy is nearly always due to the use of too small a dose. Dose is limited more by matters of cost than by toxicity levels.

*   *   *   *   *

Vitamins have been amusingly described as substances that make you ill if you don't have them. More correctly, they are substances essential to certain life processes but which cannot be totally synthesised by the body. Thus, they must be taken in with the diet, ready made, or at very least their precursors, chemicals from which they are easily derived, must be available in the food intake.

What is to be regarded as a vitamin for one animal may not be for another. For example, mice have no need of vitamin C though other rodents like guinea pigs do, as do humans. This raises an important factor. For although mice can live without vitamin C, they do not always do so. And experimental mice who have vitamin C added to their controlled diet appear to thrive and resist disease better than those who are without it. This has considerable relevance to the whole matter of

[3] Newell, Dr. G., National Cancer Institute of America.

vitamins and vitamin deficiency states.

If an animal is deprived of an essential vitamin for a sufficient length of time it will start to display symptoms of vitamin deficiency disease. A well known example is that of scurvy that affected sailors on long voyages up until the eighteenth century. Over a period of time it was discovered that lack of vitamin A resulted in increased vulnerability to disease. Shortage of B vitamins caused beri-beri and failure of blood producing mechanisms. Vitamin D shortage resulted in the soft bones and curiously shaped bodies of rickets. Only the tiniest amounts of the relevant vitamins are needed to prevent these deficiency states.

Orthodox medicine recognises vitamins as important only in relation to deficiency disease. According to that viewpoint it is only necessary to consume the small amounts that prevent deficiency. Over the last ten years, however, it has become increasingly apparent that this is not the whole story. Contemporary, but as yet unorthodox, opinion now sees vitamins cast in a different, far more extensive role. The suggestion is that there are widely varying degrees of vitamin deficiency, as there are different degrees of severity of many other diseases. It seems likely that what is normally regarded as deficiency is really only the most severe, pre-death stage of deficiency. That can be corrected by administering the small dose that will bring the sufferer back from the brink of death. But the small dose will do no more. Work is now progressing to show that although no longer in a fatal state there is still a relative shortage, for higher doses promote even greater degrees of health and resistance.

This has given rise to the use of megavitamin dosage. In this, doses far higher than those held by orthodoxy to be of value, are administered. I am personally devoted to the practice of megavitamin therapy and have one infallible suggestion to make to doubters. Go on to a harmless megavitamin course for one month and see the difference. I seldom see anyone unconvinced by this simple personal test.

The question of relevance of megavitamins to cancer medicine is an interesting reflection on the orthodoxy versus unorthodoxy tussle. Years ago I remember professionally unqualified 'healers' (or rather, as they were then all described, 'quacks') proclaiming the use of vitamin A as a preventive and curative cancer routine. The idea was always laughed off by those of us who knew better.

Much evidence has now been accumulating to show that *we* were wrong and *they* were right. Some 16,000 cases attending a routine medical screening centre in London had some part of their blood stream samples stored. Recent re-examination of these has shown that there was no statistical relationship of blood vitamin A levels with other variables like age and smoking habits. However, vitamin A levels were considerably lower in patients who subsequently developed cancer, particularly cancers of the lung and gastrointestinal tract.[4]

So much evidence has been amassing that the *British Medical Journal*[5] recently devoted its main academic leader to a view of vitamin A relevance.

More than 75% of the vitamin A found in the average Western diet comes from retinol or similar compounds found in liver and dairy produce. The rest comes in the form of carotene or carotenoids, the molecules of which are split to yield vitamin A in the large intestine. The main sources of carotenes are carrots and green leafy vegetables. Orthodox researchers showed in 1976[6] that shortages increased susceptibility to carcinogens in the respiratory tract and the bladder. Animal experiments also show that natural retinoids inhibit or cause regression of tumours deliberately produced by chemical carcinogens.

A large trial in Norway[7], which again associated a low incidence of lung cancer with high dietiary vitamin A intake, was equalled by another in Japan.[8] In this the risk of lung cancer was found to be reduced by a half in those who had daily intake of green or yellow vegetables. A more recent trial (to be published later in the *Journal of Chronic Diseases*, by J.D. Kark and colleagues) found that those with low retinoid blood levels had a six times increased chance of developing lung cancer. Yet another report, to be published in *Nature*, by Peto, Doll, Buckley and Sporn, suggests that attempts to increase serum concentrations of carotene may prove to be more useful. It is already known that the more carotene consumed, the less is converted to vitamin A and the more enters the serum as carotene. This is probably the most important factor.

The point to be stressed is that Hans Nieper, as reported in the previous chapter, announced that publicly in England in May of 1980. Others long before him had proclaimed the importance of vitamin A and similar compounds. Yet most of today's cancer cases in the United Kingdom and many other countries are *still* not receiving, either in tablet form or as part of a planned diet, an adequate amount of vitamin A or carotene. One wonders what it needs to shake up those in authority and *insist* that this deplorable state of affairs is brought to a speedy end.

The use of vitamins of the large B group has achieved more recognition when it comes to the use of larger than the 'recommended' doses. There has long been an injectable form (Parentrovite) and this has been widely used, though largely by 'fashionable' physicians, who have discovered its value in a wide variety of conditions. Vitamin B12 (a

---

[4] *Lancet*, 1980, ii, 813.
[5] *Brit. Med. J.*, 11 Oct. 1980, 281, 6246, 957.
[6] Sporn, Dunlop, Newton and Smith, *Fed. Proc.*, 1976, 35, 1332-8.
[7] Bjelke, E., *Int. J. Cancer*, 1975, 15, 561-5.
[8] Hirayama, T., *Nutrition and Cancer*, 1979, 1(3), 67-81.

cyanide containing compound) in minute doses prevents the disease of pernicious anaemia. This disease is not uncommon in patients who have had the stomach removed by surgery (gastrectomy) for peptic ulcers. A degree of anaemia often results in post-gastrectomy patients causing a low degree of health which is often not complained about, and not recognised when it is.

Vitamin B12 has another, rather unorthodox use. It is well known that giving large doses, perhaps twenty times the 'recommended' monthly requirements, every two or three days for a fortnight or so, engenders in the patient a far higher state of well being and healthy feeling. It has an euphoriant effect that is often just what is needed to start picking up a person who has been in a low state of general health for some reason or other. This is an example of the use of an unorthodox megavitamin routine that is quite widely practised by orthodox physicians. It is another incongruity that they remain ignorant of or deliberately blind to other, similar, equally useful kinds of megavitamin therapy.

Doctors may also be rather gullible or inclined to hear what they want to hear. I have already mentioned the way in which prematurely and perhaps (but by no means certainly) unjustifiably, those wishing to promote amygdalin have allocated to it a provisional place amongst the B vitamins as B17. There has also been an attempt to place another alternative preparation, pangamic acid or pangamate, at position B15. This raised the ire of orthodox workers who regard the material as of unproven value.

Instead of setting out to prove it had no value, which might, though I doubt it, have proved possible, they tried a most questionable trick. They used it in a way it would never be used for humans, to show that, so misused, it could cause cancer[9]. Of course it can cause cancer and can be toxic. Most things can. On the other hand it is nowhere near as toxic or carcinogenic as the drugs used in chemotherapy. This unfair dodge fooled a lot of people. One of the country's leading medical journalists, Dr. Eric Trimmer, who, virtually single-handed, has been responsible for more advance in his own specialised field of Sexual Medicine than anyone, was so hoodwinked. In his column[10] he wrote that he was glad "the Americans have cracked down on vitamin B15". The Americans hadn't. Only the *Journal of the American Medical Association* and other parts of the establishment had done so. Even Dr. Trimmer, shrewd old sceptic that he is (and much esteemed by the present author), fell into the trap about the carcinogenicity.

Both sides of these controversies use deplorable and unfair

[9] *J. Amer. Med. Assoc.*, 1980, 243, 24.
[10] *Medical News*, 18 Sept. 1980, p. 30.

promotional and denigratory techniques. Everyone, professional and lay people alike, must be on the watch for the easy and competent techniques that are so able to trick us. Neither blind faith nor academic status are any substitute for an open mind.

Of all the vitamins that have received publicity in the matter of megavitamin therapy, vitamin C is by far the best known. For years, famous Nobel Prizewinner Linus Pauling has recommended its regular intake in large amounts for a number of benefits. When small town doctors and fringe medicine naturopaths recommend vitamins in doses far in excess of known physiological needs, they are likely to get laughed at. It is somehow harder to laugh at Nobel Laureates.

The first idea in modern times of using vitamin C as an anti-cancer drug came from a Canadian physician, McCormick, in the late fifties. He had noticed similarities between the microscopic picture to be observed in scurvy and the appearance around invading malignant cells. It occurred to him that vitamin C shortage could be involved in both conditions. Also it is known that cancer patients are often depleted of vitamin C, suggesting that it is used in large quantities.

Since then Pauling, in association with a Scottish surgeon Ewan Cameron, have gone much further. Their work is thoroughly described in their own book[11]. About ten years ago Cameron, having read of the theory and having decided that some of his cases were so far advanced that they had nothing to lose, started putting a few people on large doses (10 grams daily). In his own words, "they responded very dramatically indeed, being converted from a hopeless terminal, 'dying' situation into a hopeful 'recovering' situation".

Here Cameron was assailed by a problem of ethics that affects most of us in cancer treatment. If there is a suggested substance that may help, it should be thoroughly tested. That involves using it in some cases then comparing results with others who do not receive it. To many of us, however, it is unthinkable to withhold, from patients who may well have no second chance, a treatment that can give relief from pain and may well extend their lives. Cameron made his decision and treated a hundred cases. When compared with other cases from hospital files, he concluded that there was strong evidence that vitamin C alone, in megadosage, had extended the lives of his patients by an average of almost a year.

When others who did not believe the theory, and who consequently were not aware of any ethical problems, tested the routine, they did not achieve the same result. The reason, Cameron and Pauling believe, is that most of the cases tested had already had cytotoxic drug treatment, whereas for the most part Cameron's cases had not.

[11] Cameron and Pauling, *Cancer and Vitamin C.* Linus Pauling Inst. of Science and Medicine, California, 1979.

This raises a most important matter. There are a number of instances, and vitamin C treatment is one of them, in which so-called 'alternative' treatments work less well, or not at all, in patients who have already undergone orthodox exposure to radiation and, even more so, to cytotoxics.

In the case of ascorbic acid (vitamin C), this appears to be explained by one part of its three-part function. One of the repression mechanisms that restricts excessive cell growth depends on an enzyme, hyaluronidase, which normally aids such growth, being in turn kept in check by an inhibitor called PHI. This latter substance requires ascorbic acid for its own synthesis. So, vitamin C shortage means too little PHI and therefore less restriction of cell growth. Another function of the vitamin is to encourage synthesis of collagen fibres in the tissues, thereby 'strengthening' the tissue and making it harder to invade by infiltrating malignant cells. Third, and most important of all in this context, is the value of vitamin C in increasing competence of the immunological function. For example, it is known that high intake levels increase the development of white cells known as lymphocytes and raise the levels of blood circulating antibodies. If cytotoxic drugs have already been 'effectively' administered, the direct damage to immune mechanisms prevents the latter responding to the vitamin's immunopotentiation. The principle being that it's no good flogging a dead horse!

The whole sensitive matter of whether or not to try orthodox therapy first and only have a go at unorthodox methods if the former fails, is thrown into very sharp relief by this point. Quite certainly, if unorthodox methods are to have their best effects, they will largely depend on the integrity of an immune system which has not been previously impaired.

Although long term trials of vitamin C on patients will take some years to present their evidence, more scientific proofs are already available.[12]   Using tissue cultures of highly malignant tumour cells (melanoma), it was found that cells were killed by vitamin C. As the cells tend to accumulate copper ions, also held to have a lethal effect on malignant cells by some unorthodox workers, the effect is particularly powerful and, "if the results can be duplicated in humans and animals with achievable doses of ascorbate (vitamin C), the specific cytotoxic effect of the vitamin can be exploited therapeutically".

Although long neglected by health food enthusiasts and having acquired little if any significance in cancer therapy, even vitamin D is now receiving attention. Normally involved with bone growth and calcium metabolism, some physicians (Dr. Hans Nieper, for one) regard the D group as important in the production of the anti-cancer steroid

---

[12] *Pulse*, reporting *Nature*, 31 May 1980.

tumosterone.

Vitamin E has, for a far longer time, been held to be of value. Unfortunately, very little of a constructive nature has been published about its properties. The vitamin, and not all accept that it is one, is a tocopherol compound. It was discovered some decades ago that the tocopherols, when fed to mice and rats, increased their apparent sexual interest and the rate at which they accomplished copulations and attempted copulations. No tests so far carried out reliably have shown any evidence that these effects on rodents are in any way paralleled in human beings. Nevertheless, large numbers of men and women take the vitamin in the hope that it will potentiate their sexual responses.

Some of the best documented reports for vitamin E come from a leading American scientist[13]. He, like a growing number of workers, believes that much of the problem with cancer occurs at the individual cell membranes. This is the highly complex interface between one cell and another. Through the membrane not only must waste materials be removed, but oxygen and nutrients must enter. Furthermore, the membrane must bear certain sensors capable of responding to the proximity of other cells and perhaps initiating repression mechanisms to keep cells in orderly growth.

The cell membrane can be damaged in a number of ways. One such is by the influence of atoms or groups of atoms comprising what are known as free radicals. All these amount to is that they are very highly reactive, because they possess an odd or unpaired electron and are thus electrically energised particles. If the radical is able to react, it may deprive another chemical component of its completeness, leaving it, in turn, seeking something else to react with. Thus, one free radical may initiate a chain of other reactions. Should such reactions occur at the cell membrane, the electrical potential there is sure to be disturbed . . . a factor many regard as a considerable weakness.

Free radicals are common in polyunsaturated fats in the diet. They can also form as a result of exposure to radiation. Passwater regards a number of things that function as anti-oxidants as being able to combat and neutralise the radicals, thus limiting further damage and carcinogenic activity. Vitamin E is one of these, as is the mineral selenium. Supporting evidence comes from numerous sources.[14-17]

*   *   *   *   *

[13] Passwater, Dr. R.A., *Cancer and its Nutritional Therapies*, Keats Publishing Inc., Connecticut, 1978.

[14] Shamberger, R., *J. Nat. Cancer Inst.*, 1972, 48(5), 1491-7.

[15] Wattenburg, L., *J. Nat. Cancer Inst.*, 1972, 48, 1425-31.

[16] Wan-Bang Lo, S. and Black, S., *Nature*, Dec. 1973, 1322, 21-28.

[17] Franklyn, R., *Lancet*, 12 June 1976.

Enzymes play a role in practically every biochemical process known. When two pure chemicals react in a test-tube, it is only necessary for the ions of which they are composed to be mixed together for the reaction to take place. The speed of the reaction may be influenced by such things as the intimacy of the mixture, the temperature, and so on. When chemical reactions take place in the body, far more rigorous controls are required. Precise amounts of one material must react with appropriate amounts of others exactly as and when required. This is achieved largely by the intervention enzymes. Some chemical reactions will only take place in the presence of a catalyst. This is a material essential for the reaction but which does not take part in it.

The definition is true only in that at the end of the reaction the catalyst remains unaltered by what has happened around it. Enzymes are catalytic, but at least in a large number of instances they do take active roles.

The material on which the enzyme acts, its substrate, may first react with the enzyme and the resulting combination may then break down into other substances, re-releasing the intact enzyme for further use.

An aspect of biochemistry important to cancer treatment is the breaking down of protein materials. The chemical material believed so important in shielding malignant cells is a mucoid protein, mucopoly-saccharide. It is attacked and split by proteolytic enzymes, the natural source of which, in the body, is the pancreas. The main function of proteolytic enzymes, in health, is the dissolving of food material proteins into a suitable condition for absorption. Their value in de-shielding, though vital, is a quantitatively smaller role.

Enzymes can be supplied to the body in a number of ways. By mouth is a good route, the product being compressed into tablets or made into a drink. It can also be administered, if the patient has a reluctance to take things by mouth, in the form of colonic irrigation, inserted high into the rectum in the form of an enema. Another method is bladder irrigation for malignant papillomata and prostatic carcinoma. Useful enzymes are the bromelanes, derived from pineapple, such as ananase, and the commoner proteolytic enzymes or proteases. These are in widespread orthodox use for inflammatory conditions, and in fibro-cystic disease which reduces pancreas function. Their newer, far more dramatic effect, seems quite unknown to the majority of doctors.

Halstead[18] states further, that the use of enzymes is based on evidence that cancer cells are more susceptible to lysis or destruction than are normal cells when exposed to proteolytic enzymes, though he does not quote the source of this important fact. He describes a defective

[18]Halstead, Dr. B., *Metabolic Cancer Therapy*, GQ Publishers, Colton, California, 1978, p. 10.

quality of the cell membranes of rapidly proliferating cells, a contention some may regard as differing from the concept of mucoid shielding of cells. It is, however, recognised that both the blood and lymphatic fluids of young people tend to have higher concentrations of proteases than older people. There is a possible connection here with the known higher cancer incidence in older age groups.

As enzymes are of very low toxicity and are very safe to use, it does not seem necessary to await full explanations of their mode of action before using them. Some tumours which are easily accessible from the body surface can even be directly attacked with enzymes. These include breast tumours and some abdominal growths. A suitable combination of enzymes (1000 mg) dissolved in amygdalin solution (2.5 g in 50 ml) can be injected gently but forcibly into the central mass of the tumour. The usual precautions of pre-injection aspiration are required as aberrant blood vessels may occur in tumour tissue, or other vessels may have been displaced.

If injections are given at three or four day intervals there may be actual destruction in the tumour. Liquefied matter can be removed through a wide bore hypodermic needle. Removal of large amounts of tumour material in this way reduces the overwhelming effect the growth may be having on immune system resistance, and also, by diminishing tumour size, reduces the undesirable effects of any pressure it may be exerting on other organs.

With the use of amygdalin and enzymes, the degree of tumour lysis can be considerable. When it takes place there is a rise in the toxic products of lysis, currently in circulation. This can result in the patient suddenly feeling more ill and appearing to worsen. It may be severe enough in effect to warrant a diminished intensity of treatment. Patients should always know of the possibility in advance and such a temporary 'crisis' should be recognised by both doctor and patient as a good sign.

*   *   *   *   *

Minerals are the inorganic components of the earth's crust. Some, while in their single state undoubtedly minerals, are assembled into organic or living material. Common such components are carbon, oxygen, hydrogen and nitrogen. There are many others.

As a result of usage rather than accurate scientific definition, minerals tend to be thought of, medically speaking, as meaning those substances, many of them metals, which exist in small amounts in the body. A considerable number of these elements are vital for both construction and function. Perhaps the best known example is iron. Amongst other functions this is essential for the manufacture of the molecule of haemoglobin, the oxygen-carrying substance that makes blood red.

Whereas iron is needed in large amounts, as are the calcium and phosphorous essential to bone formation, many other elements are needed only in tiny quantities. Equally essential to balanced good health, these are known as trace elements. Some minerals, like sodium, are involved in maintaining the acid-alkaline state of body fluids. Others are required in minute quantities as they are vital to countless enzyme activities.

To a large extent sufficient trace elements and even supplies of the minerals needed in large amounts are obtained from food sources or dissolved in drinking water. Some minerals appear to have a significant part to play in cancer resistance and treatment. These need to be supplemented.

Nieper has draw attention to the copper fallacy. It has been noted that in many cases of extensive malignancy, the blood copper levels are very high. This has led to a tendendency to try to curtail copper intake. In fact the problem is the reverse. Copper depletion from the tissues leads to the high circulating copper levels. The aim should therefore be to increase copper consumption. In malignancy a high blood copper associated with a low zinc level demonstrates serious impairment of the immune system and that the cancer is at high speed development. Both zinc and copper must be given, but in quantities that really merit medical supervision.

Lithium was first introduced in Denmark some fifteen years ago, for use in various affective emotional disorders. Largely as a result of accidental findings, it now attracts attention as a possible adjunct to cancer management. One of the dangers of orthodox chemotherapy is the decrease in circulating white cells upon which the body relies for much of its protection against infection. Following the discovery that patients already on lithium for mental conditions appear to suffer less white cell loss after chemotherapy, a trial was carried out in France[19]. Following this a larger trial was carried out in Italy with encouraging results[20]. In spite of voices of disagreement and doubt[21], it is now recommended that lithium orotate in moderate doses of about 250 mg daily should be given in all Gentle Method programmes in an effort to stimulate immune system response.

Magnesium, in the form of magnesium orotate and ascorbate, is also required, superseding earlier use as magnesium sulphate. In general this reflects a trend for using minerals in chelated form as these are held to be more effective. Chelation merely means a chemical compound in

[19] Charron, and others, *Lancet*, 1977, i, 1307.
[20] Visca, and others, *Lancet*, 1979, i, 779.
[21] *New Eng. J. Med.*, 1980, 302, 809.

which a central metallic ion is attached to an organic molecule at two or more points.

Sodium is an essential component of many compounds found in the body. Its commonest form of consumption is as table salt, sodium chloride. So widespread is this substance that it appears as a contaminant in almost every place from which it has not been ruthlessly excluded. Some cancer therapies regard the presence of sodium as one of the main problems (see Gerson, Chapter Five), and devote much of the treatment programme to eliminating salt intake and attempting to replace it with potassium. Although supportive biochemical evidence is lacking, the experience of Gerson and many others since, shows clearly and without doubt that in the present state of knowledge salt should be regarded as probably a major factor in cancer cause and a major obstacle to its cure.

It is regrettable that over the last two or three decades there has been a huge commercial effort to supply ready-made or convenience foods of all kinds to the mass populations. It must be said that these vast masses tend, in general, to be of less cultivated palate than the higher social and intellectual strata. One of the easiest ways to make industrial food seem as if it were 'tasty' is to add salt. Over a period of time the excess use of salt has resulted in a huge proportion of the population now equating taste with saltiness. Unless food is liberally treated with salt it seems dull and uninteresting to the palate. In fact it is the reverse that is true, for salt quite efficiently masks most of the real flavours that are in food. The subtleties of natural tastes and fragrances, treated with the most delicate of cordon-bleu culinary skills, are swiftly neutralised by a sprinkling of salt.

It would be difficult to overstress the wisdom of an enormous cut in salt consumption. Only a minimum is ever required and contamination and natural content between them adequately supply this under all normal, temperate conditions. Furthermore, there is the advantage that the long assaulted taste buds will quickly redevelop their abilities and permit the rediscovery, or perhaps discovery for the very first time, of a huge range of pleasant, unfamiliar flavours.

One of the most interesting discoveries concerning minerals in the last ten years has been the hitherto unrealised value of selenium. It was noted that minute selenium traces added to drinking water of susceptible experimental mice cut their cancer incidence from 82% to 10%.[22]

Premature ageing and heart disease also appear to be reduced by adequate selenium intake. In veterinary work it was noticed that selenium in anthelmintic sheep preparations introduced in some parts

[22] Schrauzer, Gerhard, *Annals Clin. Lab. Science*, 1974, 4(6), 441-7.

of New Zealand coincided with the disappearance of sheep cancer[23]. Dr. Christine Wilson, a University of California nutritionist, drew attention to the fact that high selenium content in the food of some Asian women might explain their substantially lower rates of breast cancer. Asian diets also contain less polyunsaturated fats. This combination appears likely to be highly protective. When these women move to and adopt the food habits of Western countries their breast cancer incidence increases.

Selenium acts in at least three ways. As a component of an enzyme system (glutathione peroxidase) it inhibits oxidation of unsaturated fats and the consequent release of many free radicals. Passwater[24] also lists immune stimulation, detoxification, and antioxidant protection of all membranes as other values of selenium.

Many unorthodox physicians (Nieper, Contreras and myself included) now regard selenium as a mandatory part of treatment. Dr. Schranger, already quoted, has stated his opinion that if every woman in America now began taking a selenium supplement, within a few years breast cancer rates would decline. Many of us feel that all other cancers would decline, too, if everyone had an adequate intake.

There is no longer any reason why natural selenium sources should not be brought to their highest level by eating of wholegrains, eggs and leafy green vegetables. At the same time there should be a daily supplement of not less than 100 microgrammes.

*   *   *   *   *

The two commonest kinds of cancer are those of the lung and the large bowel. It does not need a particularly shrewd observer to note that the two areas involved are also those that are in close and continuous contact with the environment. Both skin and lungs are exposed to air but only some parts of the skin are exposed at any time, and skin is a far more resistant barrier. The delicate lungs are much more vulnerable. Thus it was not too difficult to draw the connection between lung cancer and pollution of the air that ventilates the lungs for twenty-four hours a day. The association of cigarette smoking and lung cancer was quickly hypothesised and repeatedly confirmed.

The large bowel is also in very close environmental contact. Ingested food passes quickly through the mouth and oesophagus. It pauses for a while in the stomach, which is an organ designed to accept and cope with a wide variety of incoming material. Food next passes

---

[23] Wedderburn, J.F., *New Zealand Vet. J.*, 1972, 20, 56.

[24] Passwater, R.A., *Cancer and its Nutritional Therapies*, Keats Publishing Inc., Connecticut, 1978, p. 147.

fairly quickly along the small intestine and most of the assimilable nutrients are removed from it. By the time the large bowel is reached the food bulk is much reduced and the residue awaits excretion on perhaps one or two occasions daily. This frequency is often much reduced, perhaps to as seldom as once or twice weekly.

Food material thus remains in prolonged intimate contact with the bowel wall longer than it does with anything else. These are the ideal conditions for a carcinogenic substance to have its effect. Strangely, the connection between diet and bowel cancer took a great deal longer to be spotted than that between air and lung cancer. Even now there are many who doubt the association. There are even more who try to beat bowel cancer properly without a correct diet. This is totally impossible.

With the exception of certain diseases like diabetes that are clearly in need of dietary control, it is now quite uncommon for a supervising physician to give much in the way of advice about diet to most of his cases. Yet there is virtually no case in which attention to diet is not beneficial, if not mandatory. When such advice about food is given, it is usually something vague and generalised like "Try to stick to a light diet" (whatever that is). Or "Try to eat plenty", or "Cut down on the acidy things".

This kind of unspecific advice is unhelpful and is largely ignored. Yet two or three generations ago the family doctor would not have treated a sore throat or a dose of measles without instructions about diet.

Let it be clearly understood, the association of diet with cancer, both at causative and curative level, is of supreme importance. There is no other aspect likely to have greater good or bad effects on tumour progress. The prospect of patients in cancer wards being fed a hospital diet of syrup-stewed fruits, custard, ice-cream, pastries, pies and adulterated preserved vegetables, is demonstration of the most infamous professional negligence.

In order to pass food quickly through the bowel, it needs to have a high fibre content. Yet modern food processing creates sales appeal by removing fibre. Fruit juices are filtered to make them more clear. Milled corn has the germ and husk separated. Cellulose is extracted whenever possible so that the resulting finished product shall have a soft, sludgy consistency needing no chewing. After refining, dehydrating, machine handling, packing, reconstituting, freezing and so on, the convenience foods that reach the supermarket shelves are very often nothing but 'empty' calorie containers. No wonder that they are now known as 'junk' foods.

I have no doubt that this alarming tendency, which has accelerated rapidly in the last twenty years, is thoroughly bad for general health. Warnings were given long ago, amongst others by British Medical

Research Council doctor Denis Burkitt[25]. Ex-naval Surgeon-Captain T.L. Cleave links not only cancer but ulcers, heart disease and diabetes, with overconsumption of refined carbohydrates[26].

Other important work of an epidemiological nature has also been very convincing. In 1975[27] a survey was carried out in California on the American religious sect, the Mormons. These folk have a generally moderate lifestyle, they do not smoke or drink, they have a well balanced diet with plenty of grains, fruit and meat. It was noted that their cancer rates were substantially lower, as much as fifty percent in some instances, than other Californian citizens.

It was noted too that as Mormons have such low cancer rates, and as the population of the state of Utah is about 70% Mormons, Utah has the lowest cancer rates of all fifty States[28]. Another significant point to arise for discussion is that Mormons are large beef eaters. They are reported to eat more than the average USA inhabitant. Yet when compared with another sect, the Seventh Day Adventists, who are some fifty percent vegetarian, it was nonetheless found that it was the Mormons who had the lower cancer rates, especially of tumours of the colon and rectum.

Much of what has been written about the pros and cons of vegetarianism has been written by devoted, even extremist, adherents of the practice. There is some evidence that a frugal diet is advantageous in cancer. There is little, if any, that confirms any notable benefits of a vegetarian diet. To say this, unfortunately, is to risk cries of protest from vegetarians, as if it were some kind of heresy. It is not. While the arguments are true that man can obtain all his needs (save for a little vitamin B12) from plant sources, it does not in any way follow that it is best for him to do so.

The animal world can be grouped in three dietary directions. The carnivorous eating only meats, the herbivorous eating only vegetation, and the omnivorous that thrive on mixtures of both as available. Man is admirably equipped as one of the latter. It would be ludicrous to feed a lion on grass or a bullock on roast mutton. It makes good sense for man to vary his diet to include both types.

In my quarter of a century of medical practice, I have encountered many voracious meat eaters and many vegetarians. I have not been impressed by any great differences between the general health standards of either group. Conversely, I have frequently noted a very low vitality and an appearance of only mediocre health in most vegans. Whether this

[25] Burkitt, D.P., *Brit. Med. J.*, 1973, 1, 274-8.

[26] Cleave, T.L., *The Saccharin Disease*, Keats Publishing Inc., Connecticut, 1975.

[27] Enstrom, Dr. J.E. and Austin, D.F., *Science*, 4 March 1977.

[28] Lyon, J.L., *New England J. Med.*, 15 Jan. 1976, 294(3), 129-133.

is because it is that kind of person who is drawn towards veganism or whether it is a property conferred by the practice I do not know, though I suspect both factors to be relevant.

I have also detected very often in what one might term the more dedicated vegetarians, a kind of partly concealed fear or hatred of flesh and all to do with it. In my earlier work in Sexual Medicine I frequently noted this to be associated with either a restricted ability of sexual expression or a fierce over-emphasis on sexual matters. I am left with the impression that vegetarianism is by no means always the result of logical thinking, but often results from obedience to a far deeper emotional tendency. Vegetarians should regard this as intended to be enlightenment rather than criticism.

Perhaps one should also differ from the view that holds it to be wrong to kill for food. The person who would decline to kill or eat a chicken or a fish will, however, seize living plant matter, draw it straight from the ground and devour it while still alive. If they feel that plants are so different in their qualities of life that it is more just for them to be treated worse than animals, then I reserve the right to differ.

When vegetarianism is brought into the matter of cancer nutrition there are some very important facts that need to be cleared up. First, in the early stages of treating an active malignancy that has already reached life-endangering proportions, a largely vegetarian diet is of immense value. The diet, which is discussed in detail later, should however be regarded as 'highly vegetarian but with animal material supplements'. The merit is *not* in the principle of vegetarianism but in the fact that for the ill patient, at that stage, mainly vegetable matter is most suited to the needs.

One reason sometimes given in favour of a vegetarian diet is that, as a result of its lower protein concentration, this preserves available pancreatic proteolytic enzymes. As they are not needed to digest dietary protein, more are available to attack the cancer, as earlier described. This sounds logical, but isn't.

Enzymes are mainly protein and thus high quality protein from meat, soybean, eggs and fish are valuable as sources. What is more, if protein intake is cut there would, for a short while, be a saving of enzymes. However, the body is highly efficient. Very soon after the protein intake is reduced or stopped, there is a corresponding reduction of enzyme production. The body does not go on using its limited protein supplies to manufacture enzymes it no longer needs. The reverse is probably true, that pancreatic enzyme production is stimulated by the presence of sufficient protein in the diet.

As for what should be eaten, the emphasis should be on trying to eat as much good quality, unadulterated food as possible.

An awful lot of nonsense gets talked and written about the value of

TC - H

'health' foods, 'natural' diets, and so on. A kind of vogue has grown up that suggests that that which is 'natural' (whatever that means) automatically equates with being good and wholesome. Nothing could be further from the truth. There are places where a tiger is a natural part of the environment . . . but he may eat you just the same.

That warning note having been sounded, of course there is a great deal to be said for, for example, routinely consuming a diet that is 'natural' as long as it is carefully balanced and, above all, nutritious. The spectacle of vegans devouring their nut cutlets, sprouting bean shoots and vegetable juices, then finishing off with a plate of doughnuts stuffed with synthetic cream is too bizarre for words. And it is far from healthy.

However, an ever vigilant Nature has provided us with a very reliable, if not actually quite foolproof, built-in safeguard. This is all too frequently neglected, but if used it comprises a highly protective facility. It is the combined senses of taste and smell.

Natural foods that also taste good are, virtually always, good for us. Poisonous things nearly always taste bad. Unfortunately, though thankfully rarely, a child's curiosity or adult hunger may overcome the warnings. Children are also at risk as they may copy animals and birds, thinking perhaps that these luscious looking berries they see other creatures enjoy must be alright for them too.

There is a further significance to taste. Foods containing the things we need not only look and taste good to us, they will even be found acceptable when the stomach is already full. Grapes or other fruits and nuts after a meal, for example.

From all this a hazard arises. For we are tampering with flavours on an alarming scale. Almost everyone old enough to remember what things used to taste like, agree that many of our current food supplies do have less taste now. Chickens, strawberries, tomatoes, apples, eggs and white bread are just a few. We need foods for numerous vital purposes like protein building, energy supply, combatting pathogenic intruders, and so on. We must therefore have either a degree in nutrition, or another reliable method of selection from the wide available choice. The significance of taste in this selection is unequalled. And it is now being seriously impaired by artificiality.

The nature of taste thus merits serious consideration. The earlier concept of only four basic tastes, sweet, salty, bitter and sour, is no longer tenable. At least twenty different ones are now recorded. Other things also vary the taste. Receptors at the front of the tongue may interpret some amino acids as sweet while others only produce response in more posteriorly positioned receptors. Wine drinkers will be familiar with the different flavours on the tip of the tongue and back in the palate.

Textures are relevant too, as in eating oysters. So are 'metallic' sensations found in some mushrooms. Also there are the pungent things like herbs and spices. What is more, astringency probably deriving from polyphenyl contents is an important component in such widely differing comestibles as apples, teas and wines.

Odours, as in the bouquet of wines, are often more than mere smells. They are taste-active and activating. Or things may be of almost non-existent odour but delicious taste, like oysters and beer. They may even have an unpleasant smell while amply fulfilling the needs of taste. The 'strong' cheeses like Pont L'Eveque and Roquefort belong here. In general, however, smell is the initial screening process. For badly smelling foods tend to be seldom tasted.

Until recently there have only existed two ways of artificially changing or producing non-natural flavours, and thereby dodging the taste-smell selection system. One of these, fermentation, is a natural process, though it is harnessed unnaturally by man. Not only more unusual things like sauerkraut depend on fermentation. It is easily overlooked that all beers, wines, spirits, cheeses and, of course, breads are products of fermentation in some controlled process or other.

The other variation which is totally unnatural is cooking. Delightful and subtle the result may be in creating the endless variations of different flavours heated together. But the dangers of this artificiality are there too. Cooking totally destroys some vitamins and some amino-acids. And some products of grilling and barbecueing are known carcinogens. Vegetarians frequently step in and point out that cooking renders inedible or scarcely edible foods, like meats, palatable . . . something they include as a danger. Man's 'naturally' omnivorous digestive capacity they may or may not accept as relevant.

But now there are far greater dangers. Modern methods of food production really are a cause for concern. We now eat almost nothing that is natural. The 'natural goodness of farm-fresh' produce really does have a hollow ring. For a start there are practically no natural strains of plant or animal being grown. They have been selectively eliminated and replaced by man-made strains in the interest of yield, appearance, long shelf-life, and so on. Andalusian peasant onions bring tears to your eyes; nursery grown onions can be eaten like apples.

Here we enter the very real and fearful realm of pollution. Fruits are picked 'green' for their long storage ability. Then they are falsely 'ripened', perhaps by ethylene gas. This improves the colour wonderfully. But the natural ripening is completely absent and so are the flavours that normally come from ripening. Animals are submitted to forced growth, then killed very young. It's cheap and quick, but the 'old boiler' flavours don't have time to arrive.

Artificial fertilisers of plenty of nitrogen and a few other simple chemicals in no wise equate with the natural ecosystem of the soil. Lack of sulphur means less flavour in onions, broccoli, cabbage, and eventually less flavour in meats fed on low sulphur fodder. Significant taste losses result from absences.

Unnatural presences are also an increasing problem. Chemical sprays that 'loosen' oranges for easy picking introduce 'non-orange' tastes. And countless new tastes enter foods with the chemical compounds of pesticides and preservatives, many of whose names are unknown to us, like dalapon, heptachlor . . . and, of course, DDT, which is forbidden in some western countries but widely used in other countries that produce our foods. One can only imagine the new potential for cooks, heating up a medicated chicken, with a little aldrin, some synthetic onions and a spot of 'butter-yellow' coloured cooking fat!

To be deadly serious, what emerges is that our own selective and protective taste system evolved over vast times in a natural ecosystem. Now, inside one or two generations, that entire system is thrown into upheaval. We may well be losing the safety factor of taste.

Taste, smell and sight *do* manipulate appetite and consumption. They can't work when they are tricked by their own genetic and conditioned responses being blinkered or confused by substitutes. It is the 'healthy' things like fruit, grain and vegetables that are most subjected to intruding influences. And sooner or later nearly all of our thousands of chemicals enter the food chain and land on the plate.

The significance of taste in disease is already being investigated[29]. Specific taste changes in the form of cravings or revulsions are well known in some conditions of the body harbouring a 'growth', notably pregnancy. Researchers have suggested that such cravings represent 'the body trying to tell us something'. Once again, desire and taste are important guides. Emphasising the adage that a little of what you fancy does you good, I have always found it profitable to recognise and encourage such tastes in relation to food.

It is a regrettable complication of many illnesses that they tend to curtail appetite. This is very much the case with malignancy. Except in stages of acute illness, this should always be combatted by an adequately nutritious diet. Weight loss must be regarded as unacceptable. Even when there is no desire to eat, the patient must use some willpower and eat anyway. Supplies cannot be adequate if, as a mistaken kindness for the patient, they are restricted to a few milky drinks and easy to chew and swallow morsels of junk. Cancer patients can and do waste away from malnutrition. Such inadequate nutrition brings further weakness and vulnerability to infection.

So, in cancer the patient must eat. If he or she is too weak for that

[29]Brewin, T., *Lancet*, 1980, ii, 907.

then the relatives must insist on hyperalimentation or intensive intra-venous feeding, such as has already been successfully tested in orthodox cancer treatment[30]. This can and does very often bring a patient back from the brink of death and can win time for a resumption of more thorough treatment. It is stressed, however, that this kind of parenteral feeding must be in the form of amino acids, fats, some carbohydrates and supplementary vitamins, minerals, enzymes, and amygdalin admin-istration. It is criminal neglect to think that an intravenous drip of dextrose-saline (sugar and salt) such as is often used to combat surgical shock, is a satisfactory substitute. Such a drip is poisonous and is as likely as not to be fatal. With the sole exception of an emergency treatment of dehydration, it should never be used on any cancer case in any circum-stances. And it is certainly not hyperalimentation.

The best cancer diet, as a principle, should be high in protein, vitamins and supplements, and low in carbohydrate. The importance of this has been pointed out by Dr. Dean Burke, a man who after thirty-five years of work in the highly orthodox American National Cancer Institute, grew disillusioned with its failure and turned to unorthodoxy as the only hope.

It is, in my opinion, not so much a matter of what you eat, but that it should be of nutritious quality, natural and unadulterated content, and that it should have an adequate balance of everything required. Such a diet is the Bio-Diet, which is given in detail later.

*   *   *   *   *

Increasing importance is now being attached to the question of allergy as a carcinogenic factor. Allergens (or antigens) which constitute intruding 'non-self' material are combatted in the body by specific anti-bodies. In this normal sequence there is no cause for concern. But some people overreact to one or more allergens. Their reaction is far more fierce and there is release of another chemical of the histamine type. This produces a variety of symptoms from the raising of skin wheals or blains, to irritation, swelling of mucous membranes, respiratory distress and even death from anaphylactic shock.

The aspect of allergy related to cancer causation is believed to lie in the prolonged irritation of the allergy sufferer. Far more people than has hitherto been realised live in more or less continuous states of chronic allergic response. If, for instance, a person is sensitive to milk protein, the reaction is life long. If the sensitivity is discovered and obvious milk products are removed from the diet, the reaction may still continue as

---

[30] Copeland, E.M., Report to Clinical Congress, American College of Surgeons, San Francisco, 14 Oct. 1975.

small but adequate amounts of milk are used in countless other foods, and thus repeatedly enter the body.

A more recent discovery has been that of allergy addiction. This is a state in which the sufferer is, consciously or not, addicted to the very substance that causes the unpleasant reaction. Many such allergens are consumed in small amounts perhaps several times daily. Discontinuing them may produce unpleasant withdrawal symptoms, though fortunately these are of short duration.

Whether or not the association between allergy and carcinogenesis is eventually proved, it is clearly wise for any person to discover any possible allergies that might be affecting him or her. As inhaled, or surface applied allergens tend to be less common and are usually detected anyway, it is swallowed allergens that comprise the bulk of the problem. Anyone who has the slightest suspicion of suffering from an allergy, or who would like to undergo a test to find out, can carry out two simple and most informative home routines for the purpose.

The first is a preliminary test and should be regarded only as a useful guideline. It is not intended as a substitute for skilled medical care in cases of severe allergy. It is given in far greater detail in a book on the subject by the inventor[31] . The principle of the test is that the pulse rate is raised by allergen-containing foods. Although prone to many errors, it is a very worthwhile test. Both tests are here described in the form of giving actual instructions.

First, you make a routine of taking your pulse for at least a whole minute and recording the rate, numerous times each day for several days. The times must include before rising, a few minutes before each meal, three times at half hour intervals after each meal, and just before retiring to bed. All measurements are taken in the sitting position. At the same time as all this is going on, you record every item you eat and when. If you can stick to a simple diet of a limited number of things, this will produce a far more clear picture.

This easy technique is quite capable of picking out a single bad offender. (A man whose pulse rate went shooting up and who got a severe headache after eating a chocolate mousse was just one case I recall.)

Next step is to make single food tests, for a few days if possible. At about hourly intervals throughout the day you eat a small portion of just one food. Pulse is taken before and after. The items chosen should be those most commonly eaten (bread, sugar, butter, milk, jam, cabbage, potato, meat, and so on). Any food producing an increased pulse rate should be tested on subsequent occasions.

The other excellent test is similar in some ways but more drastic.

[31] Coca, Dr. A.F., *The Pulse Test*, Arco Publishing Inc., New York, 1979.

It does not involve pulse counting. If you can, you should fast completely, allowing yourself only mineral water for a day or two. If you can't manage that then allow yourself one food only, say natural orange juice or well washed apples. After this period much of whatever allergens you had in your body should have been eliminated and any symptoms should have subsided or disappeared.

You then start on what has been called the Cave Man Diet. You are allowed only a few items of the simplest types of food that might have been available to a cave dweller. Select perhaps five items, beef, carrots, wholemeal bread, apples, hazel nuts. For the next two days you may eat as much as you like, but only of items from your list. If there is a sudden return of unpleasant symptoms, suspect one of the five items and test them carefully. Over the course of two or three weeks, increase your dietary spectrum by two or three items only, every two or three days, carefully watching for the slightest onset of symptoms. If and when you find a suspect food, eliminate it again, totally, for several days, then challenge yourself with it again. If it is a culprit, it will upset you each time.

A large proportion of people who never even suspected themselves to be allergic will detect personal kinds of poisons by these two tests. Many find themselves subject to immensely improved health just by eliminating one or two problem foods. Anyone detecting such an allergy should also have professionally done extra tests to assess the extent of the problem and to seek possible desensitization routines. Others may happily be able to exclude the causative factor easily and to their great and continuing benefit.

*   *   *   *   *

If there is one thing that makes its impact more and more clearly, the longer one works in the field of cancer therapy, it is the extreme importance of mental, spiritual and emotional aspects. The significance of these factors in the causes of cancer has already been pointed out at some length. Here the main concern is their relevance in therapy, both preventive and curative.

I will declare my position at once, which is that I am firmly convinced that any or all of these factors are of great relevance in many cases. Some people have the kind of minds and faculties that can be turned against their disease and towards the uplifting of morale. Other, simpler folk may lack this capacity, but may still be capable of influence by very helpful outside encouragement from others. This still leaves a proportion unlikely to be aided at a mental level. This does *not* mean that they are doomed, or even that they will do less well in treatment. It simply means that they lack the benefits of one particular weapon.

They may very well more than make up for this deficiency by a better than average response to some other aspect of treatment. People are different, and one of the great advantages of the Gentle Method is that it can be suitably tailored to individual needs, with infinite variety, as long as certain basic principles are maintained.

A major problem in cancer therapy is always the degree of fear that is encountered. Whatever the physician says and however hopefully books like this one are written, most people have now seen something at least of cancer, probably at close quarters, as it is now so common. The horrors are widely known, as are the miseries of treatment. Few, if any, know many people who have ever survived the ordeal and returned to decent health for any length of time. Cancer consequently spells doom. And no one has done much to curtail this concept as yet.

There is another unpleasant aspect to the fear which is frequently encountered. Few speak of it openly but, having noticed it sufficiently often, I find that an element of it can quite often be detected by gently probing questions. This is the concept that in some way a diagnosis of cancer is a re-payment, a punishment for some past error. Indeed, in some ways there is no doubt that it is. Errors of judgment leading to faulty lifestyles increase cancer proneness. But this is not the way the punishment is interpreted. The phenomenon is far less prevalent in Eastern religions than it is amongst Christians and Hebrews. This may well be the negative effect perhaps, not so much of religious belief, but of theological interpretation in the early impressionable years. Acceptance of the idea of a jealous god, the wrath of god, the sins of the fathers being visited on the children, and so on, is, I believe, important constructional material in the building of the misdeed-and-punishment concept. Although I personally do not regard the concept as genuine, there is no doubt that it exists and no doubt that it acts against the better medical interest of the patient.

This is not necessarily so of all religion. Where religious beliefs are strong, and where they are positively rather than negatively orientated, they can most certainly work for the patient. They can combat despair, set examples, and yield comfort. Also, while conviction of the existence of a better life hereafter seldom induces anyone to hurry and get there, that idea too can be consoling to someone who feels death may be near.

Religious argument can also be used to reinforce therapeutic measures. The human mind most certainly has a huge potential capacity to help in malignant disease. Every available scrap of this must be used. It is important to encourage or, if necessary, try to instill into the patient a very certain will to live. As part of this promotion it is interesting to ask a patient just why he or she wants to overcome the disease and go on living. The answer usually given is that it is because of the needs of the children, the family, or even the patient's chosen work and other responsibilities. These reasons are all good enough in themselves.

What a patient usually does not express is any purely selfish wish simply to stay alive and get healthy and well again. They probably have such selfish thoughts, but for some reason it appears morally unseemly to declare them. It is not. In fact it is most important to develop as powerful as possible an individual, honest, and selfish wish to continue life. It is entirely wholesome to want to live, just for oneself alone. This is the very fundamental level of the self-preservation urge which is currently rather unfashionable but which is in everyone, and which is so desirable an adjunct to cancer treatment. Religion can come to the aid of a believer here, when it is pointed out that self-love is both permitted and encouraged rather than the reverse by both Christian and Hebrew religions. If self-love is, as I believe, a manifestation of the selfish and desirable will to live, then it is in every way to be fostered. It may be as well to point out that in the Old Testament (Leviticus 19:18), it says quite clearly, ". . . thou shalt love thy neighbour *as thyself*". It is widely held that the main object of this teaching is the feeling of love for others. Be that as it may, it clearly says "as thyself". This implies that the degree of self-love is a considerable quality. And this self-love is not in any way deprecated.

Furthermore, in the New Testament too (Matthew 19:19), when Jesus was asked by the young man of great possessions how he might have *eternal life*, the sixth piece of advice given was to repeat the words ascribed as being spoken by God to Moses. "Thou shalt love thy neighbour *as thyself*". (My italics in both cases).

Nowhere has the value of mental capacity been greater applied to encouraging a strong will to live than in the work of the American doctor Carl Simonton. His ideas and methods have been mentioned earlier. Like much unusual, pioneering work if it comes from a member of the medical profession, Simonton's work has been extensively criticised. Much of it has indeed been anecdotal, mere stories of successful cases. Such are also to be found in this book, though it is stressed that their value is in no manner statistical, merely as examples of what can and does happen.

The basis of Simonton therapy is that patients can learn actively to participate in their own treatment. The diagnosis of cancer usually sounds like a death knell. Thereafter, patients feel that they no longer have any control over events. They feel obliged passively to accept the decisions and procedures of their doctors in what will be the final stage of their lives. This encourages a negative attitude of low resistance. When the Simonton method teaches these people that those who participate positively really will feel better, live longer and, later on, if need be, lay down their lives with dignity, it comes as a revelation. It is usual for the idea to be accepted with great enthusiasm.

A word of caution is in order. It is wrong to place too much responsibility on the patient. This is especially true of emotional support techniques like Simonton's visualisation, meditation and hypnosis. The patient is to be an active participant, yes. The patient is to realise that personal efforts of many types will improve the chances of life and health, yes. But the patient should never be made to feel in any way responsible for failure or for slow success rates. Needless guilts and false hopes should *never* be induced in any patient by any doctor for any reason. They are always wrong.

A cancer sufferer is ill. It is unwise to place too great a load on any one who is ill. Genuine hope and steady encouragement aided by specific techniques are the rule. Over zealousness is counterproductive and is one of the reasons why the balanced approach of the trained physician, when correctly applied, does better than the exuberant enthusiasm of a devoted lay healer.

Similarly, delving too deeply into the past for explanations is rarely beneficial. Everyone who looks back can find possible stresses that might have influenced cancer growth. This does not mean that they did. Neither do such incidents necessarily mean the patient should feel guilty, either for causing the stress by some misdeed, or for being unable to overcome the stress, thereby leaving himself open to cancer and his loved ones to consequent suffering. There are far too many gaps in our knowledge so far, for any specific cause and effect delineations. Thus, all ideas of guilt and punishment must be pure academic guidelines perhaps, but premature as far as any value to the already suffering patient is concerned. The Gentle Method of treatment must learn from the past, but must be totally devoted to the future in its application.

Every facet of emotional support for the patient, whether as encouragement of his or her own abilities, or instilled from without, must be aimed at showing that there is to be no question of being regarded as lost, treated as terminal, and abandoned to all but a little kindness. Rather, the patient will become the focus of an all-out team effort. The entire aim was admirably described in another book on cancer.[32]

> "A battle is on. The aim of the battle is to make however much of life remains, a pleasure and a fulfilled enjoyment. The battle itself is to be thoroughly relished and enjoyed too, as an intensive campaign against a despised and disgusting enemy. Eventually death comes to everyone, of course. But death should not be granted the honour of being regarded as a frightening defeat. At its very worst death is

[32] Bryant, I., *Cancer: The Alternative Method of Treatment*, 1980 (see Appendix).

only the end of a splendid, well-fought battle. To those of spiritual convictions it is not even that . . . it is a stage of promotion in a continuing life.

So there must be no accepting the idea that cancer is an ever-triumphant disease. It isn't. There must be no recoiling in horror at the diagnosis. No cowering in helpless fear. There must be a ruthless headlong attack on every front. The battle must be joined brimful of confidence and determination. Cancer is to be ridden down, fought to a standstill, cornered and destroyed like a wild dog. The mind and body together are well capable of this kind of combat."

The Gentle Method relies on conducting this combat by assembling every naturally existing method of offence and defence into one campaign in which they are amplified to the maximum and used synergistically.

Just before Christmas 1980, Spike Milligan wrote a most sensitive and thoughtful article[33] that had resulted from his appalling experiences during his wife's illness and death. She had had breast cancer. In his writing, Milligan had much to say in criticism of the kind of medical attitudes and inhumane treatment his wife had received. His words make grave reading. Whether or not his admonishments seem fair to doctors is beside the point. It is that the doctor's actions and words seemed wrong to the patient and her husband that is important. When one doctor, who had previously seen his wife, declined to give further advice as she had refused his medicine, Milligan reminded him of the fact that "some men take the Hippocratic Oath and then hide behind it". That doctor's callous act should, irrespective of the circumstances, send a shiver down anyone's back. It is a warning to all those who practise medicine.

But in his article Milligan says one thing of great importance. "Except in extreme circumstances, I see no point in telling a person with terminal illness that they are going to die." I agree totally with that statement. But, and it is a big but, there is a considerable span of time before any case can, or should, be regarded as terminal. Indeed, one can never accurately assess a case as terminal except in retrospect. Now, before it is genuinely terminal and thus, by definition, totally hopeless, the fight still continues. If Mr. Milligan, instead of 'terminal' means 'diagnosed as cancer, even in a late stage', then I do not and cannot agree. At all stages before terminal, there is still a battle on, for life perhaps, certainly for improved health and certainly for an extended span of worthwhile life.

Now, for that battle to be fought at its best, and by all, it is

[33] *Doctor*, 18 Dec. 1980, 10(49), 14.

extremely valuable for the patient to know exactly what is being faced. There is never any indication for sudden, brutal confrontations with unpleasant truths. But the patient can and will fight harder and better when in possession of the knowledge that it really is a fight for life, not a foregone conclusion. In the cases with which I am concerned I always pay great regard to the views and feelings of friends and relatives. After all, they know the patient better than anyone and their information and help is vital. Usually they see the point when it is explained.

I do not like to see my armamentarium deprived of even one weapon, especially such a powerful one as the patient's willful fighting spirit. I think that in most cases this is unleashed all the greater when the patient is in full possession of all the facts. Then it is a question of up-sleeves and get on with the job. British people in particular, I find, tend to have this attitude.

A number of serious workers in the cancer field have failed to recognise, or have even denied, the relevance of mental aspects of aetiology and therapy. This is strongly in evidence in those involved in research and who work in large hospitals or institutions. Mental qualities are notoriously difficult to quantify and reduce to tables of comparable figures. Just because suitable methods of measurement have not been devised does not mean the methods don't exist of course. Radio waves existed, unsuspected by the entire previous population of the earth, long before there was a population and before there was a system of artificially creating, receiving and measuring them. At least the existence of the possible relevance of mental factors in cancer should thus be accepted.

The experiences of doctors in the big organisations are sure to differ from those in close contact with individual patients. Where the doctor may not even know the patient's name and may speak of her to a nurse as 'that woman in the third bed', there may well be efficiency in terms of cost-effectiveness, number of cases seen, and so on. But this kind of medicine will not work in a great number of instances, as it deals with cases, not with people. Where the "Rent-a-doc" system operates, and patients are just so many 'contacts' and computer printout microdots, the emotional features of disease will invariably be missed.

Of course this system does not work in improving overall health. This is made manifestly clear because in spite of the advances in medicine, taken as a whole, people simply are not getting better. Even in the United Kingdom, where every kind of service has been available, and free for over thirty years, there are longer waiting lists now than there were ten years ago. And they are not all due to greater powers of diagnosis. They are longer because more people are presenting with ill-health symptoms.

It is arguable that a placebo effect operates from a method

employing 'fighting-spirit' encouragement. Far from being a reason against such a method, it is strongly for it. Every advantage is to be seized with relish in cancer medicine. It is more likely, though, that there may well be greater than mere placebo effects operating through the neuro-endocrine and immune systems. Our knowledge of this is very limited indeed so far. Breast cancer has already been correlated[34] with the high serum immunoglobulin (IgA) of the habitual anger suppressors. It is quite certain, too, that whether or not fighting spirit extends life span, absence of hope shortens it and vitiates its quality.

The final summary that emerges is that although the precise importance of mind and the precise value of psychotherapy in cancer disease has not yet been conclusively proven, there is quite enough convincing evidence to reveal its strong influence. Once again, as one cannot afford to relinquish the value of any weapon, that alone is quite sufficient to ensure the integration of emotional amplification techniques like visualisation, meditation and hypnosis, into the Gentle Method.

*   *   *   *   *

BCG is the abbreviation by which is known an attenuated or weakened strain of tuberculosis bacteria (Bacillus, Calmette and Guerin). It is the material widely used for many years in inoculation against TB. This safe introduction of an active antigen induces the immune system to produce antibodies. This kind of stimulation of the system is therefore considered to be beneficial when the function of the system is inadequate. It is certainly inadequate where there is progressive malignant disease or this latter would have been effectively eliminated.

The danger lies in a possible overloading of an already beleaguered immune system. For this reason BCG should not be administered to a very advanced case or when the patient already feels very ill. It should also only be given after the immune system has been previously supported by administration of enzymes, vitamins and amygdalin. After this stage, when BCG is given, the onset of a brisk reaction (inflammation at the injection site) is a hopeful sign of an active immune system and thus of a good prognosis. The absence of reaction suggests the reverse.

In some conditions it has long been recognised that the injection of immunoglobulins has strong therapeutic effects. These proteins are anti-bodies produced in and extracted from the bloodstream of host animals. They can be given where there is need swiftly to raise resistance to possible threatening disease. An example is to try to prevent German

[34] *Lancet*, 31 March 1979, p. 707.

measles in an unprotected woman exposed to it during early pregnancy. Where there is concern that the immune system is in danger of being overwhelmed, some unorthodox physicians now give immunoglobulins as routine.

*   *   *   *   *

Unless the use of amygdalin, naturally extracted vitamins, and the vegetarian aspects of diet, are regarded as strictly 'herbal' remedies because of their plant origin, then herbal medicine has, until now, not featured very strongly in the unorthodox approach to cancer. That may well be about to change.

One of the few herbal substances that has maintained a long association with cancer is the mistletoe plant or *Viscum album*. Mistletoe grows on a number of trees (oak, apple, etc.), and in some ways could be seen as a 'tumour', though in this instance, of a different species altogether, actually growing on and in its host. For whatever reason, it was used by the Greeks as a poison antidote, as well as by the Romans and the ancient British Druids. The famous herbalist, Culpepper, in 1633 recommended the use of the berry juice 'to mollify hard knots and tumours'.

More up to date forms of mistletoe are still widely used in Europe. Research has been carried out in Germany[35] and there is interest in the use of injectable preparations in cancer[36] in the United Kingdom. The existence of a tumour-inhibiting basic protein is claimed, and German workers have already isolated this. A homoeopathic preparation of *Viscum album* is also in use under the name Iscador. Although I have no experience of these preparations so far, I have met others (including Dr. Hans Moolenburgh) who have, and who regard them as valuable.

[35] Vester, Dr. F., Max-Planck Institut, D-9 Munchen 15, W. Germany.
[36] Seth, Dr. R., *World Medicine*, 20 Sept. 1980, p. 73.

CHAPTER SEVEN

THE GENTLE METHOD . . . THE PROGRAMME

The essence of the Gentle Method is that it is exactly that, a method of combatting cancer by using techniques which, in comparison with orthodox principles, are easy and free of discomfort. Some have claimed that the methods are non-toxic. This is something of an exaggeration as nothing is truly non-toxic. In reality, however, the materials used are of very low toxicity, and they are employed at rates and dosages in which the question of toxicity does not arise.

The method uses large amounts of some of these preparations. This is therefore sometimes a problem. It tends to be a tiresome therapy in that the patient must face repeated and frequent taking of tablets, fluids and injections. Also, injections, however carefully given, do hurt, just a little. Some patients have a very intense dislike, even a fear, of injections. For the most part a patient's reluctance can usually be quickly overcome with a combination of the no-nonsense approach and the understanding of the patient that this is a far less painful overall technique and that anyway a measure of stoicism and will power is part of the patient's own contribution to the fight for life.

During the early stages of management there is also the question of becoming accustomed to enema treatment. To quite a number of people, the enema is a distasteful and sometimes an uncomfortable process. Once again, it is something to which the patient quickly adapts. Enema administration becomes a matter of routine, and as both patient and the lower bowel become familiar with the sensation all discomfort and dislike quickly recede.

Using the Gentle Method nearly always produces an early response in the patient. There is usually a rapid decrease in pain and a progressive feeling of improvement in a number of ways. This, in itself, is rewarding and encouraging both to the patient and to those in whose care the

115

patient is being managed.

The doctors, nurses and family see a change in the patient quite quickly. The patient feels a sense of active involvement. Much of the treatment can be written out as a programme which the patient can follow without much supervision. Thus the patient's feeling of participation is further enhanced. There is an awareness that a real and whole-hearted effort is being made by everyone. The demoralising sensation of being desperately ill and more or less finished is gradually replaced by the increasing hope. With this comes a realisation that there really is an effective choice in cancer treatment. What is more, in most cases the patient quickly recognises that it is quality of life that matters most to him or her. The awareness of some of that quality beginning to return, perhaps after a period of feeling extremely ill, is yet further encouragement. It is the rule that the patient's mood as well as physical condition starts to pick up. The entire atmosphere of the patient's environment enters a new phase. It is hard to explain this situation, but I have now seen it so many times that I can, with much confidence, write that it is to be promised and expected, and will nearly always be experienced early on in treatment.

The full cooperation of the patient and family is required. If those in attendance display a feeling of morose resignation it is a strongly negative influence. It is wrong to greet the patient ten times a day with the question "How are you feeling?" Other bad influences are impatience, ill manners, or too forceful demands. The atmosphere to be encouraged is one of calm, quiet confidence. This is not always easy. The patient is ill and probably frightened. Tactless remarks and misunderstanding are all too easy. No-one should embark on the care of a cancer patient without realising that it will involve a great deal of patience, kindness and effort. Unless they can promise all those and more, they are not the best people to act as attendants.

For the patient's part, it is important that, as soon as possible, there should be full awareness of the diagnosis, of the full scale battle that is on, and of the vital part the patient is going to play in it all. The tables must be turned on the despondency and the air of inevitable failure that so often surrounds the cancer sufferer in most contemporary techniques of management. Ideally all cards must be on the table so that everyone knows where they are. There is no need for the wearying effort to avoid unfortunate remarks, to keep up false pretences, or to manufacture an artificially brave and cheerful outlook. The hope is genuine enough. The campaign will need every scrap of everyone's efforts and ability.

I should stress again at this point that use of the Gentle Method does *not* preclude the use of orthodox methods as well. There is still a great deal of misunderstanding on the part of the patients and of the medical professions. Some doctors are not prepared to give unorthodox treatment at all. A growing number will permit them and even help administer them, but only as long as they are not at the expense of concurrent orthodox therapy.

In many instances this is a great pity. Much of orthodox treatment, as I have tried to explain, is immuno-suppressant. It quite certainly drastically curtails the body's ability to combat tumour progression. But, if the worst comes to the worst, it is better to use the Gentle Method as *well as* orthodox methods than it is not to use it at all.

I would also like to stress my conviction that however and in whatever degree it is to be applied, the Gentle Method is best used under the direction, or at very least with the co-operation and guidance of a qualified physician. There are a number of reasons for this. It is characteristic of human beings who are intensely keen and devoted to an idea or a method that they can become blinded somewhat to distasteful realities. This is a problem that has been encountered by the Simontons (see Chapter Five) in their training of cancer counsellors. With a little success, which is, understandably, a heady potion, people can easily come to the mistaken belief that they are healers possessed of some remarkable gift or knowledge. They can lose some of their quality of judgement and may find ways to rationalise what are, in fact, dismal failures. Doctors are not free of this universal hazard. But, as a result of their wider knowledge of many aspects of medicine as well as their extensive experience, they are, in general, less prone to errors of this type. If a qualified doctor is not available then any sensible person or, of course, a naturopath or other unorthodox practitioner, should certainly take control. Many are brilliant, kind, wise and successful, and nothing I have said is in any way to be regarded as a criticism of them.

The Gentle Method is not the job of the highly trained specialist. Any doctor who has successfully negotiated medical school has enough general knowledge and ability to initiate and supervise management. Very little extra skill is required. As a matter of fact, many of the doctors I know, who now work in this kind of cancer treatment, began by being persuaded to try such methods on what were already 'hopeless' cases. Nothing to lose, they reluctantly agreed to unorthodox measures only to be impressed by the results. As I have said elsewhere, nothing succeeds like success, in this as in anything else.

Another advantage of having a doctor in charge is that he has access to other, possibly useful facilities. He will be able to judge when there is a need for urgent surgery and to arrange the surgeon and the hospital that he thinks best for the job. A doctor can better estimate how urgent surgery must be, or how long may be available to initiate a build-up of the patient first. He can also work closely with others of his colleagues like nutritionists, pathology experts, nurses, radiologists, and so on, and maintain a smooth and efficient liaison. Last, but by no means least, he may well in the past have earned the esteem, affection, and trust of his patient. There is *absolutely no substitute* for a capable, caring, trusted physician.

The first requirement in any patient presenting with suspected or already diagnosed cancer is a comprehensive medical examination. This is also best done by a doctor. There must be the most scrupulous examination to decide the type and extent of the disease. It is necessary to seek other, unassociated pathological conditions. The presence of diabetes, hypertension, heart disease, and so on, may well require that other forms of treatment are continued along with the cancer management. For such a situation, which is by no means uncommon, particularly in older patients, the supervision of a doctor is essential. It is also necessary to correct any small and apparently trivial bodily ailments. Where the patient's overall condition permits it, bad teeth must be treated, localised infections healed, skin conditions soothed, and so on. With such a major struggle for health about to be initiated, the body will have enough to do. A medical 'spring cleaning' is required. Also, there will be need for full blood and urine analysis to detect discrepancies and to provide base-data against which future pathological tests can be compared. For the same reason there should also be a full mineral analysis of hair.

The overall treatment, though not in any way difficult, is certainly complex. Many substances will need to be used in high dosage in order to overwhelm the malignancy. More subtle uses of such preparations may well become possible later on when further research has yielded additional knowledge. For the present, however, the Gentle Method must be applied powerfully and in widely diversified components.

There are several ways of assessing progress, and these must be watched for constantly. Not all can be expected in every case. First, and often the most dramatic, is the decrease of pain. This is noted at once from the decreased frequency of requests for pain relieving narcotics and sedatives. Curiously, it is often the attendant that notices the reduction in requests even before the patient is aware of there being any material change. In my experience, there is some degree of pain relief to be noted in between eighty and ninety per cent of patients. To be able to reduce other pain relievers, from three or four times daily doses of morphine down to perhaps a few codeine tablets within a week, is commonplace.

Almost as soon to appear is the objective feeling of being better noticed by the patient, who is usually quick to report this and be encouraged by it. There is a reawakening of the desire to converse, read, hear the radio, look through the window, and so on. There is often, too, an extremely characteristic way in which a patient will resume a previously absent interest in the future. Some of this may be due to the reduced consumption of drugs, but it is also very noticeable in cases where, although profoundly ill, the patient has had little pain and therefore no serious amount of drugs.

An increased appetite is another frequent and early reported sign. This, in spite of the fact that in the preliminary stages of the treatment the diet tends to be restricted, uninteresting, and correspondingly rather unappetising.

Where there are surface lesions, for example in the armpit when cancerous, or more often irradiated, lymph glands have broken through the skin to form ulcers, there is commonly a marked reduction in the unpleasant odours that may emanate from them. A case of malignancy in an advanced state, in spite of the most rigorous hygiene methods, can and does often emit a characteristic odour, which is both penetrating and offensive. The patient is often not aware of this, which seems to arise from the breath, the perspiration, and indeed the skin and consequently the linen. It is noticeable to attendants on entering or even approaching the sick room, and can be detected in the corridors and stairways of large size cancer units. The diminution of this odour is not only a good sign, but is most welcome to those in attendance.

The patient soon demonstrates the possession of more energy. He or she may wake earlier, be ready for a wash or shave and a trip to the bathroom. Day-time naps reduce in duration, and conversations grow longer and less of an obvious strain. Along with this there is a marked resurgence of muscle strength. The bed-ridden patient is able to turn, sit up and adjust the bedclothes, whereas the patient who is up and about starts to take exercise and perform neglected personal and household tasks.

In the case of ulcers and other surface lesions, there is a decrease in the amount of pus that collects and the entire zone acquires a healthy or healing appearance that was absent before. As the blood and urine chemistry is periodically assessed, there are improvements in such things as haemoglobin level and white blood cell count and in other more technical indicators of all-round progress like SGOT, bilirubin and alkaline phosphatase.

A very significant sign is that if the treatment is withdrawn, or if placebos are substituted for the vitamins, amygdalin and minerals, there is a swift return of symptoms. I have no personal experience of the latter as I regard such a test as immoral. But I have read of it and believe it, as I know that treatment interruption, which is sometimes inevitable, does have this undesirable result. The reverse is also true, that there is usually a renewed remission of symptoms if a withdrawn treatment programme is re-instated. I have noticed that such a second remission often takes substantially longer to commence, is less dramatic, and may not achieve such effective proportions as did the first exposure to treatment. My advice is therefore always to start the treatment with due seriousness and only when it can be methodically continued without hindrance.

*   *   *   *   *

There are three phases of Gentle Method Therapy. One is a maintenance regime, which differs from a prophylactic routine in the degree of intensity of application. Another is the phase of strenuous anticancer therapy. The third is the routine to be used in varying degrees of emergency.

It is a fact that a large percentage of cases seeking heterodox cancer methods do so only after orthodox methods have been tried, often extensively, and have failed. Many of these are such as are normally classed as terminal or very late cases. They are usually profoundly ill from the continued effects of their disease and the treatment so far given. Commonly the immune system has been suppressed almost to the point of being ineffective. This is evidenced by a proneness to trivial infections like colds, and to the infection of surgical wounds, drains, catheters, and so on. No physician is in any doubt of the gravity of such a case. The wasted physical appearance, cachectic, sallow, hollow faced and eyed, the weakness, the demoralised spirit and absence of any humour, zest or will power is a familiar enough picture.

There is very little hope to be offered to this kind of patient. If the mechanisms on which the body relies for its defences have been smashed almost beyond repair, death should be regarded as more or less imminent. However, although hope is scant, it still does exist. The principle is to attempt to buy a little time in which to initiate support methods, and give the immune system a chance to recover. If death can be postponed, even for a few days, then more and more techniques can be introduced.

The patient, if in a conscious and sufficient mental state to understand, must be involved at once. It must be explained that although seldom painful, the methods to be adopted are strenuous and tiresome to the ill person. Nevertheless their help should be enlisted if possible. It can be promised that within days there will be improvement noted. If these days are survived, this is not a false promise. However, it is probably justified in this instance to exaggerate the degree of hope that exists. It may be a life-saving action. Again, it is stressed that the patient should know the diagnosis and that the situation is serious, though in this instance the seriousness should not be exaggerated. If there is to be a fight, it is better that it takes place with the light on so that the enemy can be identified and detected. Fighting in the dark is a bad principle.

As with all medicine, so with this advanced case first presenting for treatment. The number one rule is that there shall be no further harm done to the patient. (This dictum is part of the famed Hippocratic oath.) It means that all other treatments must be stopped forthwith.

Medication of an orthodox nature must only be permitted if there is a clearly defined indication. For example, it may be essential to continue the use of insulin in diabetics, digoxin in heart failure, and so on. Patients already on steroids can only be weaned from them gently. Narcotics may still be used, but these must be when essential and not by routine dosage. There must be no radiation or chemotherapy *under any circumstances whatsoever*. The taking of routine X-rays and the carrying out of non-vital pathological investigations must be forbidden.

The surroundings of the patient must be as bright and cheerful as possible. There can be radio, music, laughter, visits and anything else within the ability of the patient to enjoy, but never to the extent that they become an effort to tolerate.

If the patient is unconcious or moribund, intravenous feeding should be initiated by drip. The drip must contain essential amino-acids, emulsified fats, carbohydrate and vitamins.

Except for this, food intake is stopped. The only permitted intake apart from medication is of natural, unsweetened orange juice and spring water taken ad lib. Providing the patient's condition permits it (and such is not always the case in advanced malignancy), a fast is continued for about three full days. This permits the liver to catch up on its onerous task of eliminating accumulated toxins.

At the same time the liver is stimulated by the administration of a caffein enema every three to four hours. The enema is prepared as follows. Three tablespoons of ground coffee (not instant) are added to two pints of water, boiled for about three minutes then simmered for a further fifteen minutes. After straining it is allowed to cool to body temperature. An enema jug can be used with a rectal tip, or a bulb-type enema syringe. The entirety of the coffee solution is inserted slowly into the rectum and should, if possible, be retained for up to half an hour.

The rectal route is very important at this stage in treatment as it is necessary to keep up a continuous barrage of medication. As the oral route easily makes the patient nauseated it is only used for nutrients, vitamins and minerals.

Vitamin A is given in large overdose. Three or four glasses a day of freshly prepared carrot juice provide a considerable amount. Where supplementary doses of beta-carotene are not available, vitamin A itself is used. On the first day the dose is 50,000 units (one very small tablet). The next day the dose is doubled to 100,000 units and similarly redoubled on each of the next three days. At the end of the first week, the dose should be about one million units daily. This dose is only reduced when symptoms of overdose appear. These, headaches, and a tendency to yellowing of the skin, are not dangerous, and as long as dose is reduced as soon as they appear they are an excellent guide to dosage. Medical supervision of this part of the treatment, as for most of the emergency phase of the entire programme, is clearly advantageous and is to be in every way encouraged.

The dose of other vitamins is as follows:—

Vitamin B1 (thiamine), 100 mg, 1 t.d.s. (three times daily) for three
    weeks then 1 daily.
Vitamin B2 (riboflavine), 10 mg, 3 t.d.s. for three weeks then 1 t.d.s.
Vitamin B3 (nicotinic acid), 100 mg, 3 t.d.s. for three weeks then 1 t.d.s.
Vitamin B5 (calcium pantothenate), 50 mg, 3 t.d.s. for three weeks then
    1 t.d.s.
Vitamin B6 (piridoxin), 100 mg, 1 t.d.s. for three weeks then 1 daily.
Vitamin B15 (pangamic acid), 50 mg, 3 t.d.s. for three weeks then
    1 t.d.s.

An excellent high potency vitamin preparation, Parentrovite, containing vitamins B1, B2, B3, B6 and C, can be given by intramuscular or intravenous injection if the oral route is unacceptable for any reason. This can present difficulties if the muscle wasting has reduced the availability of injection sites. It is also a painful injection intramuscularly, unless given extremely slowly. The dose is two pairs of ampoules every four hours for three days, thereafter reducing to two pairs daily. A syringe containing two pairs of ampoules should take not less than five minutes to inject if discomfort is to be kept to a minimum. It is not necessary to give vitamins by mouth as well as by injection as long as the recommended dosage is maintained by whatever combination of routes is used.

Vitamin C should be given at doses of about thirty grams daily, either as tablets, powder dissolved in fruit juices, or by intravenous injection. As this is an acidic preparation orally, it can cause gastric disturbances at high dosage. If it does, the dose can be reduced or given by injection.

Vitamin E is taken, by mouth, in doses of 1000 mg three times daily for ten days, then reduced to 500 mg daily until all danger is held to be passed.

Enzymes are administered in any or all of three ways. By mouth the combination suggested is Bromelane, 4000 mg, four times daily, half to one hour before meals, and pancreatic enzymes (Chymoral or similar) at a total of 200,000 units, also four times daily before meals. Other excellent alternatives from the available range of enzymes are Wobe-Mugos, Retenzyme and Intenzyme in doses recommended by manufacturers. (For sources see Appendix.)

In cases where the tumour is accessible to a hypodermic needle, it is possible to inject directly into the mass of the growth. This procedure is only to be carried out by a competent physician. Up to 100 ml of a solution containing 1000 mg of enzyme and 2.5 g of amygdalin can be used, depending on the size and nature of the tumour, at weekly intervals.

Administration of enzymes by the rectal enema is very useful if the oral route is not acceptable. Ideally the enema is given in high dosage but low volume, for example Wobe-Mugos 1000 mg in 50 ml water, last thing before sleep and, if possible, retained throughout the night. As long as the patient is amenable, one or two similar treatments should also be fitted into the daily routine.

Doctors experienced in the management of cancer find that the rectal route not only spares the oral route but, as there is direct absorption and transport of the medication (enzymes, caffein and so on) directly to the liver via the portal system, it is quicker and more efficient at stimulating that organ. In practice, too, this technique does appear more beneficial.

A large spectrum of minerals should be given if possible, but as these too may overload the dosage feasibility of the patient some minerals have priority. These are, in order of importance, as follows:—

Zinc orotate	300 mg daily
Copper orotate	300 mg daily
Potassium, as Ruthmol or potassium citrate	300 mg daily
Selenium	500 microgram daily
Lithium orotate	500 mg daily
Iodine	0.2 mg daily
Magnesium, as orotate	300 mg daily
Iron, as orotate	1000 mg daily
Calcium, as orotate	1000 mg daily

Of this list the first five items are essential. Quantities can be split into twice or three times daily doses and are best given with or after food.

Amydalin (Laetrile) is started at once and in large doses. It should preferably be given by the intravenous route. Intramuscular injection will suffice but is too slow to be the route of choice. Test doses are given at the rate of 1.0 g on the first day, 2.5 g on the second and 5.0 g on the third. Reactions are rare but may occasionally include slight nausea, headache or shivering. Such uncommon side-effects seldom last more than an hour or two and nearly always ease after the first half dozen injections.

Following satisfactory test dosage, full dosage is commenced on day four with 7.5 g to 10 g of amygdalin intravenously, in one or two doses each day. No special procedures are required as long as standard intravenous procedure is observed. Injections should be slow, taking about three minutes to complete. This high dosage is continued for three to four weeks and is relaxed only when the patient's condition justifies it in the opinion of the doctor.

Once the initial fast period has been completed, intensive nutrition is commenced. In general the diet should be in strict accordance with the aims of the Bio-Diet explained later. It is essential that the patient consumes a highly nutritious diet even if the appetite is poor. In cases where there is reluctance, gentle but firm nagging is in order. It is important for the patient to maintain body weight and gradually start to increase it. Much of the requirement can be given in the form of liquids as these are often more welcomed by the patient. Although they sound unpleasant, particularly so the liver drink to vegetarians, they quickly become acceptable. Anyway, it should be stressed that as they are not mere food but a positive part of the therapy, they must be consumed.

1. Green drink. This is made of more or less any well-washed green leaf vegetables available. Lettuce, cabbage, beetroot tops, watercress, endives, celery, parsely, mint, turnip tops, etc. Any variety of herbs, or a little onion or garlic for flavouring. To make, put a large handful of the vegetables into a slow-speed blender with two cups of water or one cup and a large juicy apple. Blend thoroughly, strain and drink fresh.

2. Vita drink. Use any combination of celery, turnips, carrots, cucumber, radishes, cabbage, onion, peppers, potatos, tomatoes, beetroot (par-boiled), swede, parsnip; add pears and apples to taste. Place up to about 2 lb of carefully washed vegetables in the blender. One ounce of pressed olive or sesame oil is added. Add some predigested vegetable protein (or amino-acid) preparation, and half a cup of mixed grains and nuts. Blend thoroughly for several minutes. Add ice cubes and continue to blend until the texture of the product is suitable for drinking.

3. Liver drink. Blend half a pound of fresh, small size ox, calf or venison liver with half a small onion, two large carrots and two large apples. Strain or press and drink at once, or, refrigerated, within forty-eight hours.

As carrots feature strongly in the diet, remember that they may contribute substantially to the vitamin A intake. Adjust the latter accordingly and be on the watch for overdose symptoms as already described.

This intensive early application of the Gentle Method is a life-saving procedure. In view of the complexity of the regime it does place some strain on the patient. The extent to which it is pressed must be as high as possible, though always within what the patient can tolerate without being overwhelmed. This is a matter for careful clinical judgement.

Both patient and attendants should be aware in advance that this emergency regime often produces dramatic results, not all of which are pleasant. In spite of pain reduction and increased well-being in the first few days, there may well be some rapid destruction of tumour tissue.

If this happens, there may well appear a kind of toxic crisis. Circulating breakdown products may be sufficient to produce a subjective worsening of the patient's condition with onset of nausea, pyrexia and general malaise. Being prepared for this in advance largely obviates alarm. Furthermore, most people are aware of the likelihood of having to get worse before getting better, and they should also be told to regard such an interval, should it occur, as a sure sign that the treament is working.

Reactions of this type can be very severe and sudden, but are always temporary. Depending on severity, the physician should diminish the dosage programme and the overall intensity of therapy. Amygdalin and enzyme dosage is stopped while nutrition, vitamins and minerals are maintained. After twenty-four hours, amygdalin and enzymes are resumed at a 20% dosage. Further daily increments of 20% bring the dose back to normal by the sixth day. It is the patient that matters, not the treatment. Treatment should *never* be pressed so strenuously that an already precarious hold on life is in any way further jeopardised. That being said, skilled management should not find it difficult to control elevated toxicity levels by reducing then re-intensifying therapy in accordance with the overall clinical picture.

* * * * *

It is difficult to state a length of time for which the emergency regime is maintained, as it will vary a good deal from case to case. Depending on how ill the patient is to start and how rapid and effective is the response, this phase is usually continued for between three and six weeks. There is no definite end to the period. Dosages reduce gradually, diet expands, and supplementary regimes are introduced to the programme as a progressive routine. There is thus a gradual change from the emergency procedure to the phase of what might be termed strenuous application of the Gentle Method.

When this has been established, the therapeutic programme will be as follows.

Vitamin dosage remains well above the 'recommended' amounts (see table on page 126).

Enzymes are only slightly reduced. Dosage continues as Bromelane 400 mg three times daily, and pancreatic enzymes 200,000 units also three times daily, as previously, taken about an hour before meals. The enzyme enema of small volume is still given before retiring for retention throughout the sleeping hours.

A caffeine (coffee) enema continues to be given twice daily. Minerals do not decrease in dose. If the previously given list has not been administered in its entirety the amounts are increased to achieve the stated levels as soon as the patient is able to accept them.

Vitamin	Chemical or other name sometimes used	Main dietary sources	Daily requirement
A	Beta-carotene Retinoids	Liver, carrots, apricots, peaches, eggs	20,000-50,000 units
B1	Thiamine		100 mg
B2	Riboflavin	Nuts, beans, yeast, wheatgerm	30 mg
B3	Nicotinic acid/niacin		300 mg
B5	Calcium pantothenate		150 mg
B6	Piridoxin		100 mg
B15	Pangamic acid	Rice, bran, wheatgerm	150 mg
C	Ascorbic acid/ascorbate	Sprouts, oranges, lemons, green peppers	10 g
D	Calciferol	Liver	500-1000 units
E	Tocopherol	Leafy green vegetables, wholegrains	400-800 units

Amygdalin continues daily for at least four weeks at 7.5 g. If and when the patient's condition shows sufficient improvement, occasional days can now be left out, progressively, until dosage reaches 7.5 g on alternate days only. On the days when no injection is administered, an oral amygdalin in tablet or powder form is given at a dose of 0.5 g three times daily. On these days vitamin C intake is reduced to 2 g daily, the vitamin being taken at intervals as widely spaced between amygdalin doses as possible. For example, amygdalin at 8 a.m., 2 p.m. and 8 p.m., and vitamin C 1 g at 11 a.m. and 5 p.m., respectively. These timings can be varied to suit the patient's individual routine, but it is important to adhere to the principle in order to minimise the chance of hydrolysis of amygdalin which might result from taking both preparations at the same time.

*   *   *   *   *

As the patient progresses towards a more extensive food intake, a particular dietary regime is initiated. This applies at whatever stage the patient wishes, whether it be during the later 'emergency' level of treatment or subsequently. The three dietary drinks already listed should continue, and other foods are added according to wish or taste. The need to maintin body weight and a high standard of nutrition continues without let up.

The principles of nutrition, or, as it has been termed, super-nutrition[1] is that of the regime known as the Bio-Diet. The fundamental basis of the Bio-Diet, or life diet, is in accordance with the long held naturopathic view that human life and health is best maintained by consuming foods which are near to being fresh and 'living' themselves, as is possible. It is not necessary to become a health food fanatic. Nevertheless there is no mistaking that the kinds of foods that occupy high status in the Bio-Diet are to a large extent those that have become associated with health food concepts. It is one of my personal sources of amazement and concern that the value of diet in cancer management has not only been, so far, largely ignored, but even ridiculed by those in medical authority.

Correctly maintained, the Bio-Diet means that every meal is a cancer treatment. Another axiomatic way of expressing the principle of the diet is that one should eat living things to live and dead things to die. There is growing and convincing evidence and experience that diet is of major importance. It must not be ignored under any conditions.

The Bio-Diet seeks to reduce or eliminate artificial foods and food additives, and to eat as much fresh and as raw foods as possible. Of necessity this results in the preponderance of the diet being vegetarian in nature. This is not because vegetable foods are necessarily better in any other context, but because, by definition, animal matter is usually eaten less fresh, more adulterated, and invariably when it is 'dead'.

The Bio-Diet as used and taught by its major proponent in the United Kingdom, the remarkable and brilliant Norman Eddie, groups all foods under five main headings. Although there are departures here from Eddie's skilled use of the diet, the basic concept is unaltered. As much as possible of the entire intake should come from the first two groups.

1. *Bio-Genetic (or Bio-Genic).* Metaphorically speaking these are foods which represent 'stored' life or which are capable of generating life. As such, the group is largely comprised of foods which under natural conditions are the means by which life is passed on from one generation to the next. With the usual care provided by such natural processes, these life-transmitting vehicles contain the very best materials which the parent could produce from its own available resources.

All kinds of edible seeds and grains belong here. Corn, wheat, buck-wheat, sunflower, sesame, millet and nuts. Most fruits either contain seeds or are seed dispersal vehicles. In many cases the seeds are eaten as

[1] Passwater, R., *Cancer and its Nutritional Therapies*, Keats Publications, Connecticut, USA, 1978.

part of the fruit. As such these latter are to be preferred. Apples and grapes in particular can be eaten together with their contained seeds. It is only a fad to remove or leave them anyway. However, many such seeds are intended to pass through the food system of animals and survive to be dropped and to grow elsewhere. They are therefore equipped with a tough and resistant outer husk. This must be crushed by the teeth or artificially if they are to be digested. Swallowing them whole will not do. Foods of the pulse type, beans, peas, lentils, also belong in this group. As seeds are designed to survive in the dried form for long periods while retaining their dormant bio-genic capacity, it is quite satisfactory that these need not be fresh. However, many such seeds are suitable for fresh eating, but have often been ignored. Just as fresh peas and beans can be used, so indeed can fresh wheat (corn cobs), corns, nuts, and so on.

An excellent muesli can be made of components of this group:

> (To make a substantial quantity)
> Oats 2 lb
> Cracked wheat 1 lb
> Sesame seed 1 cup
> Sunflower seed 1 cup
> Barley flakes, rye flakes, bran and wheat germ, each 1 cup
> Currants ½ lb
> Black raisins and sultanas, each ½ lb
> Walnut pieces, hazel nuts, almonds (whole, chopped or
>   ground), each ½ lb.
>
> Mix thoroughly. Keep in an airtight continer. Add fresh fruit as available on day of eating and milk and/or honey to taste.
>
> *(Courtesy of Mrs. Pearl Coleman.)*

Very little animal material comes into this category. The few items are eggs, animals melts and fish roe, where this can be eaten raw. There is a curious revulsion in many people to raw animal matter. If so, animal components of this group can be left out entirely. The remarkable Dr. Ivan Popov believes that only fertile eggs have any therapeutic value. The majority of eggs marketed are sterile. He further believes, and has proved to his satisfaction, that fertile eggs can produce an as yet unisolated substance that is of particularly valuable effect. This is induced in the eggs by artificially 'stressing' them by subjecting them to movement, temperature changes, and so on. Such eggs must be consumed raw to retain their value, but sources of fertile eggs tend to be limited. For those to whom the idea is unacceptable, rather than eating the whole egg, the fertile portion can be removed from the cracked-open egg and taken either alone or mixed into some other kind of food.

Also in this Bio-Genetic group belong all of the items that can normally be eaten raw in their sprouting or germinating state. Buds and plant shoots are examples. So are corn, rice and varieties of small beans (mung, aduki, etc.). These can all be easily grown at home by a simple process. Obtain a large (up to 5 lb) glass jar. Put a large handful of beans inside. Cover the top with a piece of gauze, muslin or a length cut from a lady's stocking, and held in place by a rubber band around the rim. Half fill the jar with water and stand overnight. Next morning, drain off the water through the cover. The jar is kept on a warm windowsill. Each day pour half a cup of water in through the cover, swirl around and pour off again. In a few days the beans will swell and sprout. The entire bean and shoot is eaten, ideally in a salad. It is best to eat the sprouts when up to one or two inches long. At this stage enzyme activity is at its highest and the concentration of enzymes per given weight of sprouts eaten is maximal.

The emphasis in this entire group is on rawness and freshness. Cooking is able to damage or destroy completely, vitamins, enzymes and numerous long chain, naturally-occurring compounds.

2. *Bio-Active.* This contains virtually all foodstuffs not already in the first group, which can be eaten in the fresh, raw, or near-raw state. The less they are polluted from growing or storage chemicals the better. This means making the effort to seek out stores or producers who provide 'natural grown' foodstuffs or, of course, growing food at home. If such supplies are not available, at least surface contaminants should be removed by soaking for several minutes then washing briskly or using a brush if necessary.

From the plant kingdom comes the huge salad variety of foodstuffs, young carrots, lettuce, cabbage, celery, tomatoes, etc. Many foods normally eaten cooked can in fact be eaten raw. This is so of finely shredded cabbage, cauliflower hearts, potato, young runner and French beans, chopped or grated parsnip and swede. If cooking is essential use the nouveau cuisine method, which merely means vegetables very lightly cooked in their own juice or the minimum of water, without salt, and with just a little garlic or herbs for extra flavour.

Protein sources may need to be supplemented and this can be by emphasising the value of the pulses and by adding soy products. The jackets of potatoes are a good protein source and do not need to be cooked if they are finely chopped or ground.

Animal sources are useful too, for example in the form of steak tartare, a good quality fillet, ground at least three times and eaten raw. Liver is a positive storehouse of much that is best in animal matter, including minerals and vitamins. It should always be eaten very young and very fresh. It should not be cooked in the traditional British way, which reduces it to a black, leathery consistency. It must be cut into very thin, almost transparent slices or squares and tossed into hot olive oil for mere seconds before draining and serving.

Milk products carry a very high likelihood of being an allergic factor in many people. They are thus normally excluded from the Bio-Diet during this stage of treatment unless there is reasonable certainty that no such allergy is experienced. In this latter instance small amounts of natural yoghourt and cottage cheese can be permitted.

Honey is useful for sweetening drinks like herb teas and on the home-made muesli. Other animal contributions come from naturally raised creatures like venison, pheasant, pigeon and wild duck, and from fish taken from salt or freshwater, as long as they are not fish-farm raised. These items belong in this group only if eaten within hours of death. Otherwise they fall into the next group.

3. *Bio-Static.*   This is a substantially lower category than the previous two. Unfortunately, together with the fifth group, it forms the bulk of the modern Western diet source.

Once it has died, all previously living material, plant or animal, starts to deteriorate. Separated from the parent plant, some things, such as seeds, fruits and storage roots, may deteriorate only very slowly. Other things, green leaves and most animal matter, decay far more rapidly.

In this group belong all stored and preserved items and things which are simply no longer fresh. Root crops, potatoes, and so on, are intended to be preserved and are better than more obviously deteriorating material. All materials preserved by freezing, drying, canning, smoking, chemical preservatives and salt are, in that order, progressively lower grade components of the group. So are factory-farmed meats, and plant matter that has been submitted to high grade cropping with massive exposure to modern cultural methods including fortified foodstuffs, agricultural hormones, unbalanced artificial fertilizers and pesticides.

4. *Bio-Neutral.*   This is a group with only three types of components. Foodstuffs, the benefits of which are likely to be cancelled by their harm. Ales, beers and weak wines belong here. There is good evidence that small, regular amounts of alcohol are beneficial to a number of aspects of general health. Alcohol also has, in small amounts, a mental stimulation effect. It can also improve the appetite. On the other hand, alcohol is a liver poison. In the first few weeks of treatment it should thus be totally avoided. It can be consumed in small amounts after that, but sudden episodes of high consumption are absolutely forbidden.

Mechanically advantageous foods are the high fibre, bulk foods.

Apart from containing a few minerals and vitamins, these serve only to hasten the passage of food through the bowel. In the past they were called roughage, though for obvious reasons the name of 'smoothage' is now becoming more widely used.

Water is not a food but is still an essential part of the diet. The dangers of polluted water have already been mentioned. Water containing fluorides and high amounts of pollutants must be totally avoided. Spring and bottled waters only are permitted. These should be taken in quantities up to several pints daily because of their value in assisting the excretion of toxic waste materials. If such water supply is not available, as long as the surrounding area is not one of high pollution, rain water is an inexpensive alternative. Although it seems tasteless to start, it quickly becomes acceptable.

5. *Bio-Cidal.* The title of this group may be a slight exaggeration but it does consist of foods which quite certainly do more harm than good. Regrettably, for many people, it is a major, if not the main, source of foodstuffs. It contains all kinds of junk foods, convenience-foods and artificial rubbish; 'empty' calorie containers like refined sugar, candy and chocolate bars, sweets, jams and syrups; all items from which fibre has been removed; cakes, pies and tarts, and biscuits of all types; anything made of refined flour or rice; virtually everything artificially processed to taste soft and smooth, to be the right colour, the right shape, the most psychologically appealing pack, and so on. Pre-cooked, pre-flavoured, and preserved, these items must, at this stage, be entirely excluded from the diet.

*   *   *   *   *

There are a number of aspects of the cancer sufferer's ordinary life style that can usually be altered with advantage. One of these is to seek every possible way of reducing pollution and contamination of the environment. In part this is because of mounting evidence that many pollutants are carcinogenic. How relevant these external influences are is in much doubt. Moolenburgh regards them as highly important. Nieper regards them as far less so. Others think their main danger is as allergic reaction producers. One thing, however, is quite certain. The body has to deal effectively with all toxic materials that get onto or into it, or it will fail to survive their effects. Thus, there is a constant load placed on the elimination mechanisms and this is in direct proportion to the amount of toxins to which they are exposed. It follows that keeping pollutants to a minimum places less strain on the mechanisms. It is common sense that if these and other functions of the body are faulty, overworked, or part of an unwell organism, then the less extra strain put upon them the better. This is reason enough for strenuous, but not fanatical, efforts to minimise all such hazards.

There are a number of basic rules to follow to achieve this aim.

1. Don't smoke. Ever. Smoke from burning vegetable matter and chemicals contains many carcinogenic substances. Do not believe the propaganda that smoking is safe if you don't inhale, don't smoke the cigarette too low, use filters, use only low-tar tobacco, and so on. The risks may be reduced, but they remain a huge factor just the same. And don't believe it is smart or sexy to have a cigarette, or that you need 'something to do with your hands' when in company. The price to be paid for this kind of spurious comfort is out of all proportion. So don't allow people to smoke in your house or your presence. And don't stay in a place where others smoke. Ignore the 'Come to Cancer Country' and the 'Cool as a Mountain Hearse' kind of advertising. Leave cancer country for ever.

2. Wear natural (cotton, wool, leather) clothing.

3. Use natural sources (wood and stone) for as many building purposes as possible.

4. Use natural sources for drapes, furnishings, carpeting.

5. Avoid cosmetics unless they are free of carcinogenic oils and chemicals. Wave lotions, hairsprays, artificial skin-tan, anti-perspirants and coal-tar based lipsticks are all likely offenders.

6. Avoid aerosol material and chemical polishes and deodorants.

7. Don't live in towns or near main roads or factories.

8. Pay careful attention to water sources, avoiding drinking anything but source water, and using as pure a supply as you can for cooking and washing.

9. Pay scrupulous attention to diet as discussed above. Never consume anything declared to contain preservatives, 'permitted colouring', artificial flavours or chemicals.

Clearly parts of this list are out of the question for most people. It is therefore a matter of obeying the principles as far as they are practicable. Even in the worst circumstances it is usually possible to have one low pollution room.

Radiation is known to be a cancer-causing phenomenon. We are subjected to considerable amounts from sources like X-rays, cosmic rays, ultraviolet light, microwave ovens, televisions, digital display equipment, and even, it is now suspected, electromagnetic fields created by underground and overhead cables.

The cancer sufferer should avoid as many of these as possible. The major sources, according to the National Radiological Protection Board, of the entire average exposure are: fall-out 0.6%, occupational exposure 0.45%, disposal of radio-active waste 0.15%, natural radiation 67.6%, and medical irradiation 30.7%.[2]

Non-essential X-rays are forbidden. Their value has already been much criticised.[3] The over-utilisation of X-rays means excessive irradiation per unit of diagnostic information supplied, therapeutic impact, or health outcome. The reasons for this over-exposure are excessive radiation per film taken, excessive films taken per examination, excessive examinations per patient, lack of knowledge of the physician, undue dependence by the physician on X-rays, the physician's feeling of the need for action and certainty, and patient demand. There is, at present, a kind of faith in radiological examination which at times appears almost mystical.

Television sets should be screened with metal sheets or house bricks and watched through a mirror. Bedside digital equipment must not be within several feet. Dr. Richard Mackarness, author of *Not All in the Mind*, has detected body electricity disturbances from allergens enough to cause electromagnetic digital watches to become faulty[4]. The likelihood of an electromagnetic element in cancer, operating perhaps at cell membrane level, has already been discussed. Once again, even though concrete evidence is still lacking, repeated observation and common sense are sufficient to induce caution in exposure to all kinds of radiation.

Hygiene is important from the point of view of comfort and for removal of surface waste. It can often be combined with heat therapy by the use of saunas or long hot baths (up to an hour at 105°F) once or twice weekly. Even the weakest patient should be shaved, bed-bathed, have body orifices attended to, and so on, as a daily event.

Exercise should start on the very first day of treatment. In very ill patients it may only be possible to permit passive movements. In these an attendant gently bends and stretches the arms and legs, aids trunk rotation, and movements of the head. As soon as possible the patient must move the legs, bending one, placing the heel on the opposite knee and running it down the shin. Squeezing movements of the hands against balls of wool, flexing and relaxing the abdomen and the arm muscles, and rotation of the head, are within the ability of almost everyone. Even the gentlest exercise helps, and also preserves joint mobility ready for the time when joints will be more actively needed and used again.

Patients should be encouraged and even mildly bullied, to get out of bed, move about, visit the bathroom, and spend a little time sitting, or better still standing, to look out of the window. Stairs should be tackled, if necessary with aid, as soon as possible.

[2] *Economist*, May 19, 1980, p. 102.
[3] Abrams, H.L., *New Eng. J. Med.*, 1979, 300, 1213.
[4] Personal discussion with author, 15 January 1981.

Once the initial emergency of the detoxification stage of Gentle Method management is over, and the strenuous phase is reached, the exercise programme should be gradually increased over a period of six to eight weeks. Walking remains one of the best of exercises and when the full scale has been reached there should be not less than an hour's walking every day.

*   *   *   *   *

Attention to mental or emotional aspects of treatment is an integral part of the Gentle Method. Two main processes are used. These are meditation, and a method of self-hypnosis which also embodies techniques from or similar to the Simonton visualisation programme. Both are described here in the form of instructions to the patient as it is felt that this is the most informative method.

Meditation involves the use of a word, sometimes called a mantra, as an object of mental focus. Use a meaningless word like 'Lub-Dup' or 'Hir-Hem'. Anything soft sounding and of two syllables will do. Sit, don't lie, erect in an armchair or, if essential, propped up in bed. Place your hands and arms on the chair arms or folded in your lap. Close your eyes and try to focus them far away from you in the distance in front. Breathe in and out very gently and deeply several times. Then start repeating your mantra to yourself, out loud if you wish, though most people prefer to do it silently. Continue to repeat the mantra over and over for a period of about fifteen minutes. Don't attempt to keep your mind on it, or on anything else. Let thoughts come and go as they occur. Sometimes you are likely to 'lose' the mantra, almost as if you forget it. At other times you may just stop repeating it for a while. Don't force it, and don't chase the mantra or hunt for it if it is absent. The essence is total relaxation as thoughts flow in and out. You may feel as if you are sleeping, and may even drop off. It is unimportant whether you do or not. Throughout your meditation, whenever you think of it, you should dwell on your feeling of growing confidence and health. That is all there is to it. When you have finished, just continue sitting for a minute or two until you are thoroughly back to your usual self.

A lot of mistaken nonsense surrounds the subject of meditation. Extremists have declared it to be a way of saving the world and mankind. Idiots have stated that there is no such thing, and it doesn't work anyway. The fact is that almost everyone can learn to meditate with a daily ten minutes practice for a month or so. Once the technique is mastered, it is both pleasant, relaxing and beneficial. No-one who has not tried it properly has the right to criticise. No-one who has tried is ever does.

Of the two mind therapy methods, hypnosis is unquestionably the more relevant to treatment. This is because it is not only relaxing, but has a very strongly positive aspect to its effect. You can learn self hypnosis, correctly called hypno-auto-hypnosis, from a good hypno-therapist, or, if there is not one available, you can learn it yourself from this book or from a pre-recorded tape (see Appendix). Quite a good idea is to read the next three paragraphs softly and slowly into a tape recorder. You then play the tape back at leisure obeying the instructions as you hear them. One practice session every day for a month is ample to master the method, though benefits are normally felt long before that, usually in the first few days.

Start. "I am going to relax into a gentle, safe, hypnotic state. I will lie here on the bed, with my eyes fixed on that mark on the ceiling over my head. I will feel my body relax. My mind will remain alert. I will hear every outside sound, but unless they are important I will ignore them as they do not matter. I will be able to respond at once if there is any danger. At the end of ten minutes I will wake up refreshed and in every way normal. I will never become accidentally hypnotised.

"My eyes are now fixed on the mark. I relax my feet and all the muscles of both calves. Now my knees are relaxing ... and the muscles of my thighs, both back and front ... and the muscles in my buttocks. My eyes are still on the mark but, like the rest of my body, I feel my eyelids growing heavy and tired, still and relaxed. Now I let my fingers and hands relax and feel heavy ... and the muscles of my forearms ... and my upper arms ... back and front. My shoulder muscles relax too. Still with my eyes on the mark and growing heavier all the time, I let my tummy muscles relax completely ... and my chest and breathing muscles. My breathing is gentle and automatic. My eyes still look at the mark as the muscles of the small of my back relax, and the muscles up my spine ... between my shoulders and up the back of my neck. I feel tired and heavy all over now ... and I relax the muscles of my neck and face and even my tongue.

"Now I am heavy and relaxed all over. I will count ten slowly. When I want to I will close my eyes. As I count I will go deeper and deeper into a deeply relaxed hypnotic state of rest and peace. I will feel very safe and comfortable. One ... two ... three ... feeling dreamy and drowsy ... four ... five ... six ... getting sleepy and heavy ... seven ... eight ... nine ... ten ... deeply down now ... very deeply down ... relaxed and still and very safe."

At this point you remind yourself by saying over and over the things you want to impress on your mind. Perhaps,

"I am no longer weak and ill ... I am recovering ... improving every hour of every day ... I am getting stronger ... fitter ... healthier ... I see myself as I am ... a kind, pleasant person ... who people like ... who does good ... and who will do lots more good ... I will go on

living and doing good . . . I deserve to be healthy . . . I will be healthy
. . . I am getting better and better . . . every day . . . in every way . . .
better . . . and better . . . and better."

You then start to use the visualisation technique.

"I can look or feel deep inside myself . . . I can see my tumour . . .
it is evil . . . and dark . . . it is an intruder . . . I hate and despise it . . . it
does not belong in me . . . I will not have it . . . I will destroy it . . . my
body chemicals are attacking it . . . countless millions of my blood cells
are attacking it . . . it doesn't like that . . . it fears them . . . it should fear
them . . . for they and I are going to kill it . . . I see the vile, filthy cancer
cells being attacked . . . crushed . . . squashed . . . my healthy body is
slaughtering them as they deserve . . . and now strong . . . healthy . . .
tissue cells are growing into the dying tumour . . . pushing aside the dead
invaders . . . clearing away the rubbish . . . building a new . . . good . . .
sound and healthy body . . . I am winning . . . I am getting better . . . my
treatment, my cells and myself, we are all winning together. I feel fit and
healthy and well . . . full of strength and confidence . . . I *will* live . . . I
will conquer my disease . . . with my own will power . . . I will live long
and be strong and healthy . . . I am fit and well . . . and I will live on . . .
and on . . . and on."

After about ten minutes, when you have repeated the message and
had a few moments to relax and remember it, you say, "Now I shall
count from ten back down to one. As I do I shall grow lighter and
lighter, until, at one, I will open my eyes, become wide awake, feel fresh
and alert, and be glad that I did it. And next time it will be easier still.
Ten . . . nine . . . eight . . . seven . . . coming up now . . . six . . . five . . .
four . . . right up to the top . . . three . . . two . . . one . . eyes open, wide
awake."

Make no mistake, hypnosis works. Once you have mastered the
technique you will be able to use it not only to combat your illness, but
to help master numerous daily problems. You will be able to sleep
better, avoid losing your temper, help curtail bad habits, fears,
stammering, nervousness, migraine and other pains. You will also be able
to work and think better. In short, every day, and in every way, you
really will grow better and better.

Do not be discouraged by disbelievers and those who have tried
hypnosis and failed, or have not even tried at all. The truth of the matter
is that hypnosis is very real, and it does work. Those who say otherwise
are, quite simply, wrong.

*   *   *   *   *

As with the change over from the emergency stage to the strenuous
stage of treatment, so there is no sharp distinction between the latter and

the final or maintenance stage. Gradually with progress, treatment rates and the dosages of supplements are reduced, the dietary spectrum is widened and life comes more and more back to normal. As no one ever knows for sure what causes any particular cancer, it is never possible to declare a patient cured once and for all. The tumour may have been overcome, diminished in size, contained by defensive tissues. There is no certainty, however, that it is dead and gone forever. Furthermore, if the factors, whatever they were, that caused it in the first place, occur again, then it is not safe to say that they could not produce a new cancer, or re-activate an old one.

The only reliable advice, therefore, is that there should be constant and relentless observation. The patient should stay under his or her own careful supervision and the monitoring of the physician for the rest of life. At the same time, a sensible life style and maintenance programme should be continued also forever. This maintenance programme is, in effect, the same as the prophylactic or preventative programme, now being recommended by a growing number of workers in the unorthodox cancer treatment field.

A truly prophylactic regime should start early in life. Only in this way can bad habits be prevented. Children should be brought up on a diet similar to the Bio-Diet. Treats should not be given in the form of sweets and chocolate, but in the form of special fruit. A mental attitude is encouraged to regard junk foods as bad and unhealthy. Although children commonly go through later episodes of resistance to such teachings, the basic good ideas, once implanted, usually re-surface and prove influential.

People may often have to decide between financial and material gains, and a healthy environment. There is enough information in this book and elsewhere to help them decide to live in the country, mountain or forest areas. If health matters, there should be a natural water and food supply and a minimum of pollution.

Employment should never be sought in contaminated areas or factories. Don't become, or encourage your dependants to become, a worker in such fields as radiography, nuclear physics, or where hours must be spent before cathode ray tubes such as television, visual display units, and so on.

Basic vitamin, mineral and amygdalin intake should be kept, throughout life, at a high and protective level. The tables of dosages given on pages 123 and 126 should be halved, and are then to be regarded as permanent. Amygdalin stays at a daily dose of one 0.5 g tablet night and morning. Bromelane remains at 200 mg twice daily and proteolytic enzymes at 100,000 units twice daily taken as always up to an hour before meals.

It is stressed, yet again, that there is *no substitute* for vigilance and a consistently maintained protective regime. If only these were made, forthwith, a mandatory component of all cancer therapy, there would be a rapid improvement in the success of the entire anti-cancer campaign.

*   *   *   *   *

There are a few other ancillary techniques now available that have a prominent part to play in Gentle Method cancer management, but which can only be administered where there is an experienced physician in charge of the case. This is partly because they involve substances only available on prescription and which are safe for use only under medical supervision, and partly because they involve skills unlikely to be possessed other than by doctors.

The first of these, and undoubtedly of the highest importance, is the use of what is known as Regenerative Therapy. Several times in this volume have been mentioned the various influences that can damage the genes and bring about unwelcome changes that result in malignancy or a reduction of cell efficiency. If each new cell the body grows is to be identical with and therefore as perfect as its predecessor, it is vital that the nucleoproteins be copied with absolute precision during the process of cell division. As this does not in fact happen with each and every division, the errors in the proteins tend to accumulate.

Although the mechanism of this was not understood by him, several decades ago Dr. Paul Niehans discovered that by injecting into humans the fresh cells of foetal animal tissue, the ravages of age could be retarded. The ridicule of his profession did not stop wealthy people who could afford this costly therapy undergoing his treatment repeatedly. Nowadays fresh whole cells are seldom used as a far less expensive and less dangerous method has been developed. This relies on injecting only the active ingredient constituents of the cell nuclei. The protein RNA is responsible for, as it were, transferring the message of pattern from cell to cell. It is combinations of RNA that are now given, thus providing the dividing cell with an option of a less damaged pattern to follow. Very little scientific evidence has so far been accrued on the use of RNA but it is in wide use in many countries, including by doctors in themselves. Their experience and confidence should not be belittled. So far as enquiries have revealed, there are only a very few practitioners in this country who have experience in Regenerative Therapy. (As one of these few, the writer feels qualified to comment.)

Until now this therapy has been used almost exclusively as an anti-age treatment. Patients receiving courses of painless injections at twelve to eighteen month intervals, tell of greater resistance to infection, higher energy levels and exercise tolerance, better sexual performance, improved concentration, and so on. It is, to my certain knowledge, of my own patients, one of the two finest ways of combatting age and retaining the maximum amount of vigour in a number of prominent people who regularly have treatments. I have these injections myself and thus have no hesitation in giving them a personal recommendation. No-one who wishes to remain at the highest level of health and energy for the longest possible time should be without regular courses.

I, and a number of other doctors, mostly on mainland Europe, are now collecting statistical data. We believe that in addition to the immediately beneficial anti-ageing effects, there is another less obvious advantage. For it is our impression that in patients on Regenerative Therapy we encounter a substantially lower incidence of malignant disease. It will be some years before enough statistical data has been collected to prove this theory, but in the meantime those who wish to take every precaution against cancer, as well as enjoying the undoubted benefits of Regenerative Therapy, would do well to consider it is a routine part of their body maintenance, and if they able to find the facilities (see Appendix).

An excellent combination therapy is now available. This uses regenerative methods together with the tissue specific anti-sera originally developed by Dr. Jean Thomas, and now of expanding importance as the whole field of Therapeutic Immunology develops from its infancy into a major medical technique.

BCG vaccine was mentioned in Chapter Six. Under the circumstances discussed there it is a useful adjunct to the Gentle Method. It should be given, by injection, twice weekly for two weeks as soon as the patient's condition warrants it. After that it is given once weekly for two further weeks, fortnightly for four more injections and thereafter monthly for at least six months. On each occasion a dose of 0.2 ml is administered.

Also of value by virtue of its ability to increase the general metabolic rate is the extracted hormone of the thyroid gland. This is best given as Tabs Thyroid, 30 mg daily, rather than in the form of the more modern synthetic hormones.

Where high-pressure oxygen treatment is available, short periods of exposure can be given several times weekly. Failing this, half an hour in an oxygen tent daily or twice daily is an added advantage. The patient can help matters further whether or not oxygen is available, by having several spells a day of deliberate deep breathing. The technique is to breathe slowly and deeply at a greater rate than needed. This quickly produces the 'over-breathing' effect in which there is a sensation of fullness in the head and neck, and tingling in the extremities. It is dangerous to overbreathe too much as it can cause unconsciousness. The level should never be allowed to progress further than the earliest onset of very mild degrees of the symptoms mentioned.

CONCLUSION

OTHER MEN'S FLOWERS

This book has sought to offer for consideration, a differing view of cancer as being a result of a generalised body condition of ill health. Arising from this it has proposed an alternative method of treatment, to be conducted, preferably, as the treatment of first choice, or at least as an integral part of other methods of therapy. As author, I feel that my main contribution has been to assemble the work of others into one complete programme of cancer management, which I believe to be the best so far available. In my small garden, I have grown other men's flowers.

In proposing and explaining the entire theory, it has been necessary to disagree with much of current orthodox thinking and methodology. It is therefore feasible that accusations of iconoclasm may be levelled. To some extent such allegations have been deliberately invited for, as the author, I have considerable abundance of first hand experience of cancer sufferers, which has inclined me strongly against orthodox conduct. I have travelled widely, visited the clinics of other doctors, orthodox and unorthodox, seen their patients and known my own. I also have my own small private consulting clinic in the old town of Sandwich in Kent.

In preparing the book I have found doctors and patients to have several things in common. Traditional doctors are innured to failure, yet hopeful of a breakthrough, or they are keenly delving into experimental work for themselves. Either way, their results are very bad. Doctors converted to alternative views are, on the contrary, thrilled with early success, buoyant with enthusiasm, yet puzzled and dismayed at the reluctance being shown by their so far unenlightened erstwhile colleagues. Some are even a little frightened and are looking over their shoulders with some anxiety.

For their part, patients have in common that they nearly all die.

From these points stem my tendency to iconoclasm.

A recent study[1] was made of how women really feel about receiving adjuvant chemotherapy for breast cancer.

"No words describe the sensation . . . which starts about an hour or less after the injection. The unpleasant sensation crawls around the body. It feels as though one has had an anaesthetic that has not properly worked, only it is worse than that . . . vile." That was one woman's comment. In one group of patients studied, side effects were serious enough to interfere with treatment in 79% of the women.

It is interesting to note that the side-effects encountered were of such severity that this particular trial was stopped. The authors concluded that such therapy is only justifiable when a substantial improvement of prognosis is obtained. This shows clearly that at least here and there, even within the medical profession, responsible physicians are beginning to get the message that some of us have been broadcasting for years. The doubts are creeping slowly through.

I well remember my own conversion. A man I had known for a decade, a schoolteacher, developed lung cancer. After he had had surgery and months of treatment, I can still remember his face, when he pleaded with me, not just as doctor but as friend, not to make him have any more chemotherapy. He could not face the injections any longer, but he felt he could not refuse his hospital doctors, so he tried to work on me. He was very far gone and estimated as within three to four weeks of death. I told him what I had seen of the alternative ways of treatment, and my lack of experience. After prolonged discussion, he implored that we should have a go at it together.

We did. And he died. But he died eleven months later. And what a difference while he lived. Not only did he actually return to school for over a term, but he played golf, enjoyed his family, and grew an entire extra year's crops in his garden . . . something he declared to be the biggest bonus of all. He was active and happy until ten days before his death. I was converted. I believe that other doctors trying the method on one or two such late cases would be converted, too.

From a source I have forgotten came the saying that it is better to curse the darkness than to light the wrong candle. Such a warning could be given about the thoughts expressed in this book, but wrongly I believe. For I think that the wrong candle has already been lit, long ago, and that it has burned up enough people already.

It is my opinion that the accumulated learning and experience of an open minded physician generally inclines him to arrive at the correct conclusions. If he puts this, eventually almost instinctive, guidance into practice, even if the rationale is not yet understood, it nearly always

[1] *British Medical Journal*, 1980, No. 6255, Vol. 281, p. 1594.

turns out to be the correct action. If the doctor sees and believes that a treatment works, his judgement is likely to be right even if not understood. Furthermore, when the research into the subject finally gets done, I find it invariably bears out the doctor's clinical impression.

So, it is not necessary, and never was, to have evidence first before starting to use a therapeutic method. This backwards concept is a comparatively recent innovation derived from the ascendence of the science rather than from the art of medicine.

We must use our combined intuition and experience *now*. Then the evidence can catch up when it is ready.

Max Planck wrote that new ideas gain wide acceptance only when established authorities die. That may be all well and good for some matters. But looking around at the incessant horror of cancer, seeing people I know and care about suffer, not only from their disease but from the appalling methods being unsuccessfully used to treat them, one thing has become abundantly clear to me.

There just is not time to wait for other ideas to die out. People in vast numbers are going through unutterable horrors to their deaths. The old ideas must get out of the way. There is no point in beating about the bush. Those who hold the other opinions are wrong. They and the ideas must go.

As there are so many cancer sufferers and so many doctors and other lay therapists involved with their treatment, I am aware of the very real danger that whatever is written will appeal to some and unfuriate others . . . my own mailbag demonstrates this clearly. But I am convinced of certain things. It is pretentious of man to think he is better able than Nature to exterminate cancer. His response to the existence of malignant cells is "Kill them", more or less whatever the cost. It would be far more rational if his aim were to aid the body to do for itself the killing, that it 'knows' far better how to do.

Author and thinker Michael Wheatley put it well when he said[2] "No matter to what degree man interferes, the body itself always has to do the work of healing. Given the right raw materials, the body knows infinitely better than man how to do the job."

For far too long heterodox practitioners have been regarded as deluded, as a lunatic fringe of good people gone wrong, as outsiders. But, I pose the question, who are the real outsiders? Surely it is those who are furthest out from the truth. The truth of their orthodoxy has gone wrong, and it is the adherents of orthodoxy that are the new outsiders. Their dominance is already being demolished and will soon be replaced by better sense. That is why I hold any iconoclasm to be justified.

[2] *A Way of Living*, Annual report for 1980.

And, who know, as often before, today's dangerous iconoclasm may be tomorrow's received truth[3]. The new and better ways *are* all available *now*. No-one can do worse from them, and most do better. As I said in my opening remarks, it is no longer premature to claim that cancer really is a beaten disease.

[3] *World Medicine*, Editorial, 13 December 1980, p. 5.

APPENDIX ONE

USEFUL ADDRESSES

Information on Alternative Cancer Therapy:

> Health for the New Age,
> Trustee, Lt. Col. Marcus McCausland,
> 1a, Addison Crescent, London W14 8JP

> Cancer Help Centre,
> 7, Downfield Road, Bristol

> Kent Private Clinic,
> Sandwich, Kent, CT13 9DL

Amygdalin supplies and Vitamin supplies:

> Cantassium Ltd.,
> 225, Putney Bridge Road, London SW15

Enzyme supplies:

> Armour Pharmaceutical Co. Ltd.,
> Hampden Park, Eastbourne, Sussex, BN22 9AG

Wobe Mugos, Retenzyme, etc., and Liquid Protein Food Supplement:

> C. P. Rahlstedt GmbH Ltd.,
> P. O. Box 73 05 27, D-2000, Hamburg 73, West Germany

145

Hypnosis Tapes:

Dipix Distributions Ltd.,
Gusta Lodge, Worth, Nr. Deal, Kent, CT14 0BY

Regenerative Therapy, and Gentle Method (supervision only):

Kent Private Clinic,
Sandwich, Kent, CT13 9DL

APPENDIX TWO

SUGGESTED FURTHER READING

Cancer, the Alternative Method of Treatment, by Dr. Isaac Bryant
Roberts Publications, 225, Putney Bridge Road, London SW15.

An End to Cancer, by Dr. Leon Chaitow
Thorsons Ltd., Wellingborough, Northants.

Cancer and its Nutritional Therapies, by Dr. Richard Passwater
Keats Publishing Inc., New Canaan, Connecticut, USA.

Laetrile Case Histories, by Dr. J.A. Richardson
American Media, P.O. Box 4646, Westlake Village, Ca. 91359, USA.

A Cancer Therapy, by Dr. Max Gerson
Totality Books, Del Mar, California, USA.

A Way of Living as a Means of Survival, by Michael Wheatley
Corgi Books, 61-63, Uxbridge Road, Ealing, London W5 5SA.

Live to Be a Hundred, by Dr. Dick Richards
Roberts Publications, 225, Putney Bridge Road, London SW15.

147